Layout and design by:
Alain Sauzay - Villefontaine (38)

Original title: ***Mémento homéopathique – Du symptôme à la matière médicale***
© CEDH International Paris 2004 ISBN 2-91566-801-9

Translated from French by Bénédicte Clément
Proofread by Sheila Adrian

ISBN 2-91566-817-5

HOMEOPATHIC
MEMENTO

From symptoms to materia medica

Work done through the Institut Boiron by:

Marilyne Busser, Pharm. D.
François Chefdeville, M.D. and coordinator
Jean-Marc Cousin, M.D.
Philippe Desobeau, M.D.
Joseph Lambert, M.D.
Jean Merckel, M.D.
Josette Nouguez, M.D.

CEDH

PREFACE

Clinical practice in homeopathy is demanding, and choosing the right medicine often implies several "return trips" between patients, symptoms, and materia medicas.

This shuttling back and forth requires great experience, a top-quality materia medica and adequate and reliable tools.

The book *Homéopathie: Les Relations médicamenteuses*, published in 1998, incites us to shuttle from the materia medica to the patient to revisit clinical observation, in order to better individualize the choice of medicines and examine potential complementarity.

The "*Memento*" helps with the return journey: from a sensation, a modality, a unique symptom, it invites us to go back to the materia medicas to locate a symptom in each medicine's rich pathogenesis or proving.

If for experienced physicians this new book from the CEDH is a memento, for beginners it will be a precious guide for discovering and better understanding the far-reaching dimensions of the materia medicas.

Because of the quality and reliability of the work done by the "Materia Medica Commission", this "Memento", along with *Homéopathie*: Les *Relations médicamenteuses* and *Pharmacologie et matière médicale homéopathique*, represent essential tools for physicians in clinical homeopathy.

Jacques BOULET
Director CEDH

SUMMARY

INTRODUCTION

For physicians, many issues can arise from a homeopathic consultation, including the issue of a finite capacity for memorizing. How many times have we searched for a medicine's name since the symptom or modality expressed by the patient is in this medicine's proving or pathogenesis? We all know that an answer exists, but where do we find it, and is it reliable?

Take several examples. A patient reports salty-tasting saliva. This evokes a homeopathic medicine, but which one? NATRUM MURIATICUM of course, and maybe SEPIA, but what about LYCOPODIUM? Another patient complains about either watery yellowish fecal matter, or discolored stools that float: Do we know that the only medicine which corresponds to both of these is CHELIDONIUM? If our patient usually sleeps deeply, we think of OPIUM or NUX MOSCHATA, but would we also think of NUX VOMICA or PULSATILLA? And when patients have foul-smelling sweating of the feet, SILICEA automatically comes to mind; but do we realize that there are dozens of other possible options? When treating food cravings and aversions, especially craving for sugar, SULFUR (SULPHUR), ARGENTUM NITRICUM, LYCOPODIUM occur to us; but what are the other reliable medicines for this symptom? If patients are hungry, before or during migraines, will we know which medicine to suggest? And if at the end of a check-up we note that a patient is in better shape at night than in the morning, how can we choose the appropriate treatment?

The answers to these questions can be found, of course, in the various existing **repertories**.

The first repertory, by Hahnemann, was written in Latin and edited in 1805 in Leipzig, followed by one by Jahr (1835). Next, encouraged by Hahnemann, Boenninghausen (1845) published one, which is valuable for its **psychosomatic approach**. Many other repertories exist: Hempel (1859), C. Lippe (1879), Lee (1889), Knerr (1896) and others.

The best known, still today, is the James Tyler Kent repertory (1900), based on those by Lippe and Lee. Its vision widely differs from previous repertories. In fact, Kent applied the philosopher E. Swedenborg's ideas, mainly that spirit and matter derive from a common original substance, with the corollary that there is a mandatory psychic origin to all diseases. His repertory consequently has a **psychosomatic tone**. For choosing the right medicine, Kent prioritized symptoms, starting with: mental symptoms, cravings and aversions, general symptoms, general modalities (local modalities being secondary) and lastly local objective symptoms, considered as "common" thus useless. With all due respect to Kent and his materia medica, it seems impossible, and contrary to Hahnemann's experimental spirit, to adhere to his so-called homeopathic philosophy, which is in fact simply borrowed from Swedenborg's conceptions. This type of repertory has a number of risks linked to it: failing to diagnose serious diseases; or because of the ranking applied, trying to use homeopathy to treat something it cannot. It could also involve a one-sided psychosomatic view, or lead to the use of homeopathy by non-physicians, with all the underlying consequences. Other repertories were published in the twentieth century such as Boger's (1937), or those of Barthel and Klunker (1973-1978), which compile the works of sixteen authors (including the repertory of Kent, those of Knerr, Boger, Jahr, Allen's Encyclopedia, the new medicines from Mezger, Julian and also Hahnemann's *Materia Medica Pure and Chronic Diseases*...) in three languages. There is also the Broussalian repertory (1992) which completes Kent's repertory.

Computerized repertories which came out in the last few decades (Broussalian or Bachellerie for the French) are not guarantees of reliability because, as J. Jouanny said in the introduction to *Homéopathie: les Relations médicamenteuses* (1998): *"If you put rotten food in a freezer, it will still be rotten when thawed; it is the same with a computer: no matter what the software, it will only spew out the unreliable medicines previously keyed into it."*

The history and ideas involving the repertories allow us to point out a certain number of facts because, as varied as they may be, these repertories have their limits.

Some have remained unchanged since the beginning; others were modified or appended like Kent's. Some are simple compilations of previous repertories with added comments by their authors or others, the goal being to reach a certain symptomatic exhaustiveness, like Barthel and Klunker's repertory. In general, over the years, the number of symptoms and medicines listed in them continued to grow with no true therapeutic validation.

Most of these repertories do not take medical progress into account, since they are more than a hundred years old. Nosology has changed significantly since Hahnemann, Boenninghausen or Kent, and biology, anatomical pathology and physiopathological concepts and medical imaging are all very important today in confirming or negating clinical observations.

These repertories are not totally obsolete when seen as tools. They can be used with discernment as databanks or reminders for difficult cases needing an appropriate medicine for a specific rare symptom as long as the choice of medicine is later validated on a series of symptoms by a reliable materia medica. They are therefore only useful if the clinical observation is complete and the nosological diagnosis precisely determined.

From a technical point of view, it is better not to privilege a patient's psychological or rare signs as recommended by Kent and others due to their philosophical beliefs. Rather (this is the CEDH position), the lesion and functional signs, the localization and modalities must be taken into account when reliable. Likewise, etiology and anatomical pathology should be included if known, and a patient's psychological state if it has changed since the onset of the disease. Finally the materia medica must be checked to ensure that it lists one or more medicines with real possibilities for the case on hand.

This type of discussion shows the need for a modern tool for homeopathic physicians. Actually, this book doesn't pretend to be another repertory because it is a **Memento**. A Memento, from a Latin word meaning "Remember", is an agenda in which we write things to remember. Therefore it is selective, by nature. This book is a reminder based on very precise criteria: clarity, simplicity, reliability and therefore usefulness. It doesn't pretend to be an exhaustive listing, which would be contrary to its commitment to reliability. Great care was taken in compiling the quality information it contains, or "signs for homeopathic usage" which are of interest to homeopathic physicians and are especially useful in customizing a medicinal prescription. This book has seven chapters: modalities and etiologies; periodicities, alternations and laterality; sensations; discharges and menstruation; food cravings and aversions; sleep and dreams; and key symptoms. We chose not to deal with clinical indication comparisons as this was already treated in our last book *Homéopathie: Les relations médicamenteuses.* It is also important to note that there are no value-based judgments in this Memento because we consider that a symptom, a modality or a sensation is either reliable or not. To obtain this result, we discussed signs at length before they were included, using the early great materia medicas (Hahnemann, Allen, Hering) and more recent serious ones like those of M. Guermonprez and the CEDH. In addition, we based this selection on our theoretical and practical experience as physicians and teachers. We took the risk of omitting certain items rather than keeping some symptoms that are described in materia medicas but never encountered in practice. However, this book contains certain clinical claims that could be called "historical" for which homeopathic medicines are justified, at least as additions to classical treatments (for example AURUM METALLICUM in treating mastoiditis). We must also emphasize a fundamental point, that a diagnosis should be made first, whenever possible, before using this memento, in order to place symptoms in context: patient and proving. We also thought it necessary to draft an introduction to each chapter of this Memento. Each introduction should be read before use, so as to correctly understand the instructions, limits and framework for each listing, since our ultimate goal is to provide practitioners with a truly useful tool, even when a few of these points remain open to debate.

François Chefdeville
Coordinator of the Materia Medica Commission
May 2004

ETIOLOGICAL SIGNS AND MODALITIES

Etiological Modalities

Hahnemann placed great emphasis on etiological signs and today we still consider them highly valuable. Modalities are on the same level, commonly defined as qualifying symptoms in terms of their improvement or aggravation under various circumstances. This is why common symptoms such as fatigue or insomnia have a real value due to their etiology or modalities. It is also interesting to note that in general neither modalities nor etiological signs have pathogenetic origins (they are not listed in T.-F. Allen's *Encyclopedia*) but rather emerge from the clinical and therapeutic usage of homeopathic medicines (*Guiding symptoms* by C. Hering).

The wording "etiological signs" seems preferable to "causalities" which is often used in its place. These are events in the larger sense (food excess, jealousy, sadness, etc.) known to trigger or aggravate morbid reactions on presumably predisposed "terrains". **Because in practice we have noted that etiological signs are often confused with aggravation modalities, it was decided to combine them in a single chapter.**

Modalities, or symptom qualifiers, are general or local.

General modalities only concern a few medicines, for example: ARSENICUM ALBUM where all levels of burning sensations are improved by heat, or BRYONIA where various pathologies are improved by immobility. It is obvious that in certain cases the modality is very important and shapes the medicine, in some ways.

Local modalities concern many medicines, and by definition only apply to one part or the other of the pathogenesis. It is interesting to study the example of PHYTOLACCA. The materia medica states that there is a worsening due to cold damp weather, and improvement due to dry weather; of course, this only concerns rheumatic pathology or ENT problems, but in no way does it concern mastodynia. The mistake would be to connect the modality to "the entire train" when in reality it is only connected to one or two of its "railroad cars". This is why, in this Memento, we specify the concerned pathology for each medicine listed next to a modality.

Sometimes, general and local modalities can be totally contradictory. One example is PSORINUM where the general modality is improvement by heat, whereas the skin pruritus is improved by cold.

When a contradiction exists between a medicine's general modality and its local modality, it is usually the general modality which prevails, especially so if this is a chronic case. This apparent contradiction is not surprising since we know that the "major" medicines, called polychrests, cover hundreds of symptoms in the initial materia medicas (Hahnemann, Allen, Hering, etc.) due to the great numbers of persons testing them. This can explain the contradictory nature of some modalities.

Over 200 years of practical homeopathy have confirmed one modality or the other, but we must remain open-minded in estimating their value. It must be remembered that modalities, although important, are not eliminatory elements for choosing medicines. In fact, if a patient has all the signs of a medicine, but without its modality or with one contrary to the medicine's proving, nonetheless this medicine probably remains the appropriate one.

AGGRAVATION MODALITIES

ACIDS (Food or drinks) : *Digestive disorders*

ALUMINA — *Vinegar, but also potatoes*
ANTIMONIUM CRUDUM — *In spite of craving*
FERRUM METALLICUM — *Also with eggs*

AIRPLANE

See TRANSPORTATION

ALCOHOL

See also BEER

ANTIMONIUM CRUDUM — *Sour wines*
CARBO VEGETABILIS — *Headache, red face after drinking wine*
CHINA (CINCHONA) — *Colitis with flatulence*
GLONOINUM — *Cephalic congestion*
LACHESIS MUTUS — *Headache*
LYCOPODIUM — *In spite of craving*
NUX VOMICA — *In excess*
SULFUR (SULPHUR) — *In excess*
ZINCUM METALLICUM — *General Modality. Associated signs: cough, headache, restless leg syndrome, nausea, shaking, dizziness*

ANGER

AURUM METALLICUM — *Violent anger*
CHAMOMILLA — *Spasms: digestive (vomiting), nervous (convulsions), respiratory (asthma), genital*
COLOCYNTHIS — *Abdominal spasms, vomiting*
LYCOPODIUM — *Headache, digestive disorders*
NUX VOMICA — *Convulsions, chills, vomiting*
STAPHYSAGRIA — *Pathologies: digestive, urinary, cutaneous … due to repressed anger*

ANNOYANCE

CHAMOMILLA — *Cough*
IGNATIA — *Cough worsened by coughing*
STAPHYSAGRIA — *Headache, cough*

ANTICIPATION of events

ARGENTUM NITRICUM — *Diarrhea, precipitation*

CAUSTICUM	*Anxiety by altruism*
GELSEMIUM	*Diarrhea, insomnia, shaking*
SILICEA	*Anxiety*

ASLEEP (Falling)

See chapter SLEEP

BATH

See WATER

BED (In)

See LYING DOWN

BEER : *Digestive disorders*

ALOE	
CARDUUS MARIANUS	
KALIUM BICHROMICUM	*Difficult digestion*

BOAT

See TRANSPORTATION

BOWEL MOVEMENT (During a): *Anal-rectal spasm*

NATRUM MURIATICUM
NITRICUM ACIDUM
PLUMBUM
SILICEA

BOWEL MOVEMENT (After a)

Anal-rectal spasm

IGNATIA
LACHESIS MUTUS
NITRICUM ACIDUM

Weakness

ARSENICUM ALBUM	*Whatever the quantity, with palpitations, trembling*
CONIUM	*And syncope*
PODOPHYLLUM	

BREAD

ANTIMONIUM CRUDUM	*Nausea*
BRYONIA	*Gastralgia*
CAUSTICUM	*Gastralgia*
HYDRASTIS	*Digestive disorders*
KALIUM CARBONICUM	*Whole wheat bread*
PULSATILLA	*And butter*

BREAKFAST (After): *Diarrhea*

NATRUM SULFURICUM	*Sometimes mood improvement*
PODOPHYLLUM	
THUYA (THUJA OCCIDENTALIS)	

BUTTER (Eructation)

See **also FAT**

CARBO VEGETABILIS
PULSATILLA

CABBAGE, SAUERKRAUT

BRYONIA	
CARBO VEGETABILIS	*Diarrhea*
LYCOPODIUM	*Flatulence*
MAGNESIA CARBONICA	*Eructation*
PETROLEUM	*Diarrhea*

CAR

See **TRANSPORTATION**

CHILDBIRTH (At)

ACTAEA RACEMOSA (CIMICIFUGA)	*Inefficient uterine contractions*
CHAMOMILLA	*Hypersensitivity to pain with agitation and screaming*
CUPRUM METALLICUM	*Finger cramping, thumb flexed inside the palm*
GELSEMIUM	*Back pain going up the spine during labor; shaking*
KALIUM CARBONICUM	*Lower back pain during labor "back labor." Hemorrhoids*
PULSATILLA	*Changing back pain during ineffectual labor*

CLIMATE (According to the)

See **SEA, MOUNTAIN, SNOWY, HEAT (HOT AND HUMID WEATHER)**

CLOTHES (Tight)

See **TIGHT**

COFFEE

CAUSTICUM	*Digestive disorders*
CHAMOMILLA	*Dyspnea, gastralgia, neuralgia, toothache, dizziness*
COFFEA TOSTA	*Difficulty falling asleep due to hyper-ideation*
IGNATIA	*Constipation*
MOSCHUS	*Constipation*
NUX VOMICA	*Gastralgia, facial neuralgia, palpitations, dizziness*

ZINCUM METALLICUM	*And stimulants in general: headaches, nausea, shaking*

COFFEE WITH MILK

KALIUM CARBONICUM	*Digestive disorders*

COLD

In general

ACONITUM	*Following a dry chill*
ALUMINA	
AMMONIUM MURIATICUM	
ARSENICUM ALBUM	*Except congestive headaches and dyspnea*
AURUM METALLICUM	*Depression*
BARYTA CARBONICA	*Except headache symptoms*
BELLADONNA	*Headache after a haircut*
CALCAREA CARBONICA	*Damp cold weather*
CAMPHORA	*But wants to undress*
CARBO VEGETABILIS	*With a desire to be fanned*
CAUSTICUM	*Pains, paresis, profuse sweating*
COCCULUS	*Nausea*
DULCAMARA	*Damp cold*
FERRUM METALLICUM	
GRAPHITES	*Except pruritus worsened by heat of the bed*
HEPAR SULFUR	
HYDRASTIS	
KALIUM CARBONICUM	
MAGNESIA CARBONICA	*Neuralgia*
MAGNESIA PHOSPHORICA	*Neuralgia*
MOSCHUS	*But needing fresh air*
NITRICUM ACIDUM	
NUX VOMICA	*Coryza after a haircut*
PETROLEUM	*And during winter*
PHOSPHORUS	*Except headache and gastric symptoms*
PSORINUM	*Except pruritus*
RUMEX	*Pruritus, cough*
SEPIA	*Except disorders of the venous circulatory system*
SILICEA	*Catching a chill due to wet feet*
TUBERCULINUM	

BATH (Cold)

ANTIMONIUM CRUDUM	
CALCAREA CARBONICA	
MAGNESIA PHOSPHORICA	
RHUS TOXICODENDRON	*Cough*
SEPIA	
TUBERCULINUM	

CORYZA (During acute)

ACONITUM	
ALLIUM CEPA	*If cold air is inhaled*
BELLADONNA	
HEPAR SULFUR	
HYDRASTIS	
KALIUM BICHROMICUM	
NUX VOMICA	
RUMEX CRISPUS	*Cough if cold air is inhaled*

COUGH (During a coughing spell)

ACONITUM	
ARSENICUM ALBUM	
CAUSTICUM	*With hoarseness improved by drinking something cold*
HEPAR SULFUR	
HYDRASTIS	
KALIUM BICHROMICUM	
KALIUM CARBONICUM	
NUX VOMICA	
PHOSPHORUS	*Cough when going from hot to cold and from cold to hot*
RUMEX	*Cough when inhaling cold air*
SILICEA	
TUBERCULINUM	

DERMATOLOGICAL (During diseases)

AGARICUS MUSCARIUS	*Chilblains*
PETROLEUM	*Eczema*
PSORINUM	*Eczema*
RHUS TOXICODENDRON	*Vesicular dermatosis*
SEPIA	*Eczema*

DRINKS (Cold)

ARSENICUM ALBUM	*Stomach cramps, diarrhea, cough*
BRYONIA	*Gastralgia*
CAPSICUM	*Chills after drinking cold water*
GRATIOLA	*Diarrhea*

DRY (Cold)

ACONITUM
ALUMINA
BRYONIA
CAUSTICUM
HEPAR SULFUR
KALIUM CARBONICUM
MEDORRHINUM
NUX VOMICA

FEVER (During feverish states)

ACONITUM	
BELLADONNA	
CAMPHORA	*But wants to undress*
NUX VOMICA	
PYROGENIUM	
RHUS TOXICODENDRON	

FOOD (Cold)

ARSENICUM ALBUM	*Diarrhea*
ALUMINA	*Eructation, esophageal spasm*
CALCAREA CARBONICA	
DULCAMARA	*Diarrhea*

HEAD sensibility to cold air

BELLADONNA	
CALCAREA CARBONICA	
CHINA (CINCHONA)	
HEPAR SULFUR	
NUX VOMICA	*Coryza after a haircut; standing in a draft*
SILICEA	

HUMID (Cold)

See **DAMPNESS**

NEURALGIA (During)

ACONITUM	
ARANEA DIADEMA	
CAUSTICUM	
CHINA (CINCHONA)	*Drafts of air*
COLOCYNTHIS	
HYPERICUM	
KALMIA	
MAGNESIA PHOSPHORICA	
MEZEREUM	
PLUMBUM METALLICUM	

PAINFUL (During affections), RHEUMATISM

ACTAEA RACEMOSA (CIMICIFUGA)	
ACTAEA SPICATA	*Pain in the small joints, particularly the hands*
AURUM METALLICUM	
CALCAREA CARBONICA	*Damp and cold weather*
CALCAREA FLUORICA	*Damp and cold weather*
CAUSTICUM	*Dry cold*
CHINA (CINCHONA)	*Facial neuralgia*

DULCAMARA *Damp cold*
MANGANUM *Small joints*
PHYTOLACCA
RHODODENDRON
RHUS TOXICODENDRON
RUTA GRAVEOLENS

TOOTHACHE worsened by cold (Cold air, cold drinks)

ANTIMONIUM CRUDUM *And when touching with the tongue*
HEPAR SULFUR
NATRUM MURIATICUM *And by chewing*
RHUS TOXICODENDRON
STAPHYSAGRIA
SULFUR (SULPHUR)

COMPANY (In) With desire to be alone

BARYTA CARBONICA *Hides from strangers*
IGNATIA
NATRUM MURIATICUM
SEPIA

CONSOLATION

CALCAREA PHOSPHORICA
IGNATIA
LILIUM TIGRINUM
NATRUM MURIATICUM *Anger, crying*
PLATINA
SEPIA *Irritability and crying*
SILICEA

CONTACT Slight

See **TOUCH**

CONTRADICTION

AURUM METALLICUM
HEPAR SULFUR
LUESINUM (SYPHILINUM)
LYCOPODIUM
NUX VOMICA
SEPIA
SILICEA

CONVERSATION

See **TALKING (While)**

COUGHING (While)

In general

ACONITUM	*Painful larynx: grasps the larynx*
ALLIUM CEPA	*Painful larynx: grasps the larynx*
ANTIMONIUM TARTARICUM	*Nervous facial tics*
ARNICA	*Cries before a coughing spell*
BRYONIA	*Trachea, head and chest pain*
CAUSTICUM	*Hip pain, trachea pain*
EUPHRASIA	*Eyes watering*
HEPAR SULFUR	*Painful larynx: grasps the larynx; cries when coughing*
KALIUM BICHROMICUM	*Tracheal pain*
NATRUM MURIATICUM	*Eyes watering*
PHOSPHORUS	*Eyes watering*
PULSATILLA	*Eyes watering*
SCILLA (SCILLA MARITIMA)	*Eyes watering*

Urinary incontinence

ALUMINA
CAUSTICUM
FERRUM METALLICUM
KALIUM CARBONICUM
NATRUM MURIATICUM
PULSATILLA
RUMEX
SCILLA (SCILLA MARITIMA)
SEPIA
VERBASCUM THAPSUS

COVERED (While being)

In general

BROMUM	
IODUM	
LEDUM PALUSTRE	
LYCOPODIUM	
PULSATILLA	
SECALE CORNUTUM	*Chronic arterial disease of the lower limbs*
SULFUR (SULPHUR)	

During acute or feverish affections

ACONITUM	
ANTIMONIUM TARTARICUM	
APIS	
CAMPHORA	*In spite of a freezing-cold sensation*
CHAMOMILLA	
CHINA (CINCHONA)	
MERCURIUS SOLUBILIS	
PULSATILLA	

Aggravation Modalities

CROWDS

ACONITUM	*With acute anxiety attacks*
ARGENTUM NITRICUM	*Afraid of crowds and open spaces*
GELSEMIUM	*Afraid of crowds*
LACHESIS MUTUS	*Suffocating sensation if physically confined within a crowd*
PULSATILLA	*By shyness*

DAMPNESS, COLD HUMIDITY

In general

ACTAEA RACEMOSA (CIMICIFUGA)	*Muscle pain*
AMMONIUM CARBONICUM	
ARANEA DIADEMA	
ASCLEPIAS TUBEROSA	*Intercostal neuralgia*
AVIAIRE	*Pulmonary as well as ENT pathologies*
BARYTA CARBONICA	*Pharyngitis*
BELLADONNA	*Headache if hair gets wet*
BLATTA ORIENTALIS	*Asthma, asthmatic bronchitis*
CALCAREA CARBONICA	*General modality: with ENT, respiratory, articular, dental, ocular problems*
CALCAREA FLUORICA	*Painful joints*
CALCAREA IODATA	*Cryptic tonsillitis*
CALCAREA PHOSPHORICA	*Painful joints at snow-melting time*
COLCHICUM	*Gout, digestive disorders*
DULCAMARA	*Highly typical general modality: painful joints; respiratory disorders: asthma, nasal blockage*
HYPERICUM	*Asthma due to fog*
KALIUM BICHROMICUM	*Painful joints*
KALIUM MURIATICUM	*ENT pathology*
MANGANUM	*ENT pathology, hoarseness, painful joints*
MERCURIUS SOLUBILIS	*Painful joints, respiratory disorders*
MEZEREUM	*Neuralgia*
NATRUM SULFURICUM	*Highly typical general modality: painful joints before the rain, depression*
PHYTOLACCA	*ENT and joint disorders*
PULSATILLA	*Pollakiuria*
RANUNCULUS BULBOSUS	*ENT disorders, inter-costal neuralgia, shingles*
RHUS TOXICODENDRON	*Painful joints*
RUTA GRAVEOLENS	*Painful joints*
SARSAPARILLA	*Pollakiuria*
SILICEA	*General modality*
SULFUR (SULPHUR)	*Painful joints*
TEUCRIUM MARUM	*Polyps*
THUYA (THUJA OCCIDENTALIS)	*Breathing, osteo-articular disorders*
TUBERCULINUM	*Painful joints, respiratory disorders*

COLD BATHS

See COLD

DAMPNESS WITHOUT EFFECT on PAINFUL JOINTS

TUBERCULINUM RESIDUUM

DARKNESS, in the DARK

Fear of the dark (In children)

See also DUSK

ACONITUM
ARSENICUM ALBUM
CALCAREA CARBONICA
CAUSTICUM
LYCOPODIUM
MEDORRHINUM
PHOSPHORUS
PULSATILLA
STRAMONIUM *Often the most appropriate*

Night terrors

ACONITUM
BORAX
KALIUM BROMATUM
KALIUM PHOSPHORICUM
STRAMONIUM

Sleepwalking

ACONITUM
KALIUM BROMATUM
KALIUM PHOSPHORICUM
NATRUM MURIATICUM
OPIUM
PHOSPHORUS
SILICEA
STRAMONIUM

Walking instability, dizziness

ARGENTUM NITRICUM *And anxiety*

DAY

See TIMETABLE

DESCRIBING ones symptoms: *cries*

PULSATILLA
SEPIA

DISCHARGE (By a SUPPRESSED DISCHARGE)

See SUPPRESSION

DRAFTS (Drafts of air)

ARALIA RACEMOSA	*Watery and irritating rhinitis*
AVIAIRE	*Respiratory pathology*
BROMUM	*If feeling hot*
CHINA (CINCHONA)	*Sensation of being cold with chills, neuralgia*
HEPAR SULFUR	*And dry cold*
KALIUM CARBONICUM	
NUX VOMICA	*Rhinitis, chills in bed if covers pushed back*
PSORINUM	*Respiratory tract*
SILICEA	*Respiratory tract, asthma, headache*
TUBERCULINUM	*Respiratory pathology*
VERBASCUM THAPSUS	*Facial neuralgia*

DRESSED (While being)

See COVERED

DRINKING (After)

ARSENICUM ALBUM	*Cough and vomiting after a cold drink; chills*
CHINA (CINCHONA)	*Bloating*
COLOCYNTHIS	*Abdominal cramps*
DROSERA	*Cough*
NUX VOMICA	*Chills with a freezing cold sensation*
PHOSPHORUS	*Vomiting once the water has warmed up in the stomach*

DRY (In dry weather)

See CLIMATE

DUSK

See TIMETABLE

DUST: *Asthma*

BLATTA ORIENTALIS
BROMUM
POTHOS FOETIDUS

EATING (After)

ARSENICUM ALBUM	*General weakness*
BARYTA CARBONICA	*General weakness*
CALCAREA CARBONICA	*Drowsiness after supper*
CHAMOMILLA	*Facial sweating*
CHINA (CINCHONA)	*Gastric fullness, in spite of eating very little*
FERRUM METALLICUM	*Gastric fullness, in spite of eating very little, spasmodic cough*

HYOSCYAMUS	*Hiccups*
LYCOPODIUM	*Gastric fullness, in spite of eating very little, sleepiness*
NUX VOMICA	*Stomach cramps and need to defecate, sleepiness, dizziness; better after a short nap*
PHOSPHORICUM ACIDUM	*General weakness*
PULSATILLA	*Sleepiness, dizziness*
SULFUR (SULPHUR)	*Sleepiness*

EATING and DRINKING (While): *Diarrhea*

ALOE
ARGENTUM NITRICUM
ARSENICUM ALBUM
CHINA (CINCHONA)
COCCULUS
CROTON TIGLIUM
FERRUM METALLICUM
PODOPHYLLUM
VERATRUM ALBUM

EATING to SATIETY (While)

See also **FOOD IN EXCESS**

ANTIMONIUM CRUDUM	*Voracious appetite: bread, pork, cakes*
CALCAREA CARBONICA	*Sweets*
CARBO VEGETABILIS	*Fats*
IPECA (IPECAC)	*Fats, cakes*
LYCOPODIUM	*Heartburn on right*
PULSATILLA	*Ice cream, cakes*
NUX VOMICA	*Spices*
SULFUR (SULPHUR)	*Fats, sweets*

EGGS

FERRUM METALLICUM	*Diarrhea, vomiting*
SULFUR (SULPHUR)	

EMOTIONS Pleasant

COFFEA TOSTA	*Insomnia*
OPIUM	*Diarrhea*

EMOTIONS Unpleasant

Agitation, anxiety

ACONITUM
ARGENTUM NITRICUM
ARSENICUM ALBUM
GELSEMIUM
HYOSCYAMUS

IGNATIA	
KALIUM BROMATUM	
MOSCHUS	
OPIUM	*Shaking of limbs after a fright*
PHOSPHORUS	*And hot flashes*

Depression

ARSENICUM ALBUM
GELSEMIUM
IGNATIA
NATRUM MURIATICUM
PHOSPHORICUM ACIDUM
SEPIA

Insomnia

AMBRA GRISEA
ARSENICUM ALBUM
GELSEMIUM
PASSIFLORA

Laryngitis

HYOSCYAMUS
MOSCHUS
SAMBUCCUS
STRAMONIUM

Red face

FERRUM METALLICUM
PULSATILLA

Shaking

ARSENICUM ALBUM	
CAUSTICUM	
GELSEMIUM	
KALIUM BROMATUM	*Generalized when something needs to be done*

Syncope

COFFEA TOSTA
IGNATIA
LACHESIS MUTUS
MOSCHUS

EXCITATION (At the slightest)

AMBRA GRISEA	*Fainting spells, fatigue, bloating*
ANACARDIUM ORIENTALE	*Fatigue*
COFFEA TOSTA	*Insomnia*
IGNATIA	*Fainting spells*
MOSCHUS	*Fainting spells*

EYES (Movements of the) and head

BRYONIA	*Dizziness*
CONIUM MACULATUM	*Dizziness*
KALMIA	*Ocular pain*

EYES (While closing)

CALCAREA CARBONICA	*Visual hallucinations*
CONIUM	*Sweating*

Dizziness

ALUMINA	
ARGENTUM NITRICUM	
LACHESIS MUTUS	*With nausea*
THERIDION	*With nausea*

FALL

DULCAMARA	*Asthma, hay fever*
LACHESIS MUTUS	*And in the spring*
LYCOPODIUM	*And in the spring*

FAT

ANTIMONIUM CRUDUM	*Pastry, pork*
CARBO VEGETABILIS	*Rancid or rotten food; eructation*
CYCLAMEN	
IODUM	
IPECA (IPECAC)	
KALIUM MURIATICUM	
PULSATILLA	*Diarrhea, eructation, gastralgia, nausea*
THUYA (THUJA OCCIDENTALIS)	

FEAR

See **EMOTIONS**

FOG

DULCAMARA	*Asthma*
HYPERICUM	*Asthma*

FOOD IN EXCESS: *Dyspeptic disorders*

ANTIMONIUM CRUDUM	*Sour foods, processed meats, pork*
CARBO VEGETABILIS	*Fats*
NUX VOMICA	*And spicy foods*
PULSATILLA	*Fatty cakes*

FRUIT Unripe: *Diarrhea*

ARSENICUM ALBUM	
BRYONIA	*And flatulence*

CHINA (CINCHONA)	*Abdominal pain caused by fruit in summer*
COLOCYNTHIS	
FERRUM METALLICUM	*With stools containing undigested food*
NATRUM SULFURICUM	
PODOPHYLLUM	*Due to an excess of fresh fruit*
RHEUM OFFICINALE	*Prunes*

FULL MOON

See MOON

FULL and NEW MOON

Voir MOON

GARLIC

LYCOPODIUM	*Flatulence*

GOING DOWN (By)

See MOVEMENTS

GOING UP (When)

ACONITUM	*Tight chest*
ARSENICUM ALBUM	*Tight chest*
CACTUS	*Precordialgia*
CALCAREA CARBONICA	*Dyspnea, extrasystole, tight chest, dizziness when going up the stairs*
COCA	*In the mountains*
IODUM	*Dyspnea*
KALIUM CARBONICUM	*Dyspnea*
NATRUM MURIATICUM	*Tired legs when going up the stairs*
SPONGIA	*Dyspnea*

HEAT (By)

All forms

Atmospheric, confined, physical warm-up, etc.

AESCULUS HIPPOCASTANUM	*Except superficial pain*
ANTIMONIUM CRUDUM	*Weakness*
APIS	
ARGENTUM NITRICUM	*Except gastralgia*
BELLADONNA	
BROMUM	*And physical warm-up*
BRYONIA	*Except local pain sometimes*
FLUORICUM ACIDUM	
GELSEMIUM	*Hot weather, hot and humid*

GLONOÏNUM	
IODUM	
KALIUM IODATUM	*Except coryza*
KALIUM SULFURICUM	
LACHESIS MUTUS	
LYCOPODIUM	*Except sore throat*
NATRUM CARBONICUM	*Headache starts as soon as the weather gets hot*
OPIUM	
PULSATILLA	
SELENIUM	
SEPIA	*In spite of shivering*
SULFUR (SULPHUR)	
SULFUR IODATUM (SULPHUR IODATUM)	

CONFINED heat in a hot room

ACONITUM	*Headache*
ALLIUM CEPA	*Rhinitis*
ANTIMONIUM CRUDUM	*Mostly radiating heat: diarrhea, nasal blockage, cough*
ARGENTUM NITRICUM	*Ocular pain, photophobia*
COCCUS CACTI	*Cough*
DROSERA	*Cough*
FERRUM PHOSPHORICUM	*General state*
KALIUM IODATUM	*Nasal blockage*
LILIUM TIGRINUM	*Palpitations, syncope*
NATRUM CARBONICUM	*Dizziness*
PULSATILLA	*General state*
SELENIUM	*Headache*
SPONGIA	*Cough*
TABACUM	*Nausea*
TUBERCULINUM	*In spite of shivering*

COUGH when coming into a room, going from cold to hot

ALLIUM CEPA	
ANTIMONIUM CRUDUM	
BROMUM	
BRYONIA	
CAUSTICUM	
COCCUS CACTI	
NATRUM CARBONICUM	
NATRUM MURIATICUM	
PHOSPHORUS	*And when going from hot to cold*
PULSATILLA	
SULFUR (SULPHUR)	

COUGH worsened by heat (Hot room)

ALLIUM CEPA	
ANTIMONIUM CRUDUM	*Going from cold to hot*
APIS	
BROMUM	*Going from cold to hot*

BRYONIA	*Going from cold to hot*
COCCUS CACTI	
DROSERA	
DULCAMARA	
IODUM	
IPECA (IPECAC)	
KALIUM SULFURICUM	
LYCOPODIUM	
NATRUM CARBONICUM	
PULSATILLA	
SENEGA	
SPONGIA	
TUBERCULINUM	

DRINKS (Hot)

LACHESIS MUTUS	*Pharyngitis, digestive disorders*
PHOSPHORUS	*Headache, gastralgia*
PULSATILLA	*Headache*

FOOD (Hot)

LACHESIS MUTUS	*Dysphagia, gastralgia*
PHOSPHORUS	*Gastralgia, sweating while eating hot and drinking hot*
PULSATILLA	*Gastralgia*

HEAD (When warmly covered): *Headache*

IODUM
LYCOPODIUM
PHOSPHORUS
PULSATILLA

HOT AND HUMID WEATHER

BROMUM	
GELSEMIUM	*Hay fever, flu syndrome by hot and humid weather*
IODUM	
IPECA (IPECAC)	*Asthma due to south wind*
KALIUM IODATUM	*Painful joints*
LACHESIS MUTUS	
NATRUM SULFURICUM	
PODOPHYLLUM	*Diarrhea*

PAIN (Burning local)

APIS	*With pinkish edema*
BELLADONNA	*With local inflammatory syndrome*
CARBO VEGETABILIS	*Varicose ulcers*
PHOSPHORUS	*Nausea when putting hands in warm water*
SECALE CORNUTUM	*Arteritis*
SULFUR (SULPHUR)	

PRURITUS (Due to heat of bed)

See **PRURITUS** in the **SENSATIONS** chapter

SUN (Heat of the)

See **SUN**

THROAT pain worsened by local heat

APIS
LACHESIS MUTUS
PHYTOLACCA

TOOTHACHE worsened by hot food and drinks

CHAMOMILLA
COFFEA TOSTA
LACHESIS MUTUS
MERCURIUS SOLUBILIS

HEIGHTS (When high up): *Afraid of heights, vertigo*

ARGENTUM NITRICUM	*Feels like jumping*
CALCAREA CARBONICA	

ICE CREAMS, iced foods and drinks: *Digestive disorders*

ARSENICUM ALBUM	*Diarrhea, abdominal, gastric pains, vomiting*
BRYONIA	*Gastralgia*
IPECA (IPECAC)	*Nausea*
PULSATILLA	*Headache and nausea*

INHALING DEEPLY

BELLADONNA	*Cough*
BRYONIA	*Thoracic pain, cough*
CONIUM	*Cough*
KALIUM CARBONICUM	*Chest pain, cough*
RANUNCULUS BULBOSUS	*Intercostal neuralgia, shingles on chest*
RUMEX	*Going from a hot to a cold place, cough*

INHALING of FRESH AIR

NUX VOMICA	*Burning sensation in throat*
RUMEX CRISPUS	*Cough*

INTELLECTUAL EFFORTS

AGARICUS MUSCARIUS	*Tics, shaking, behavioral disorders, dizziness*
ANACARDIUM ORIENTALE	*Headache, irritability, gastroduodenal ulcer*
ARGENTUM NITRICUM	*Dizziness*
ARSENICUM ALBUM	*With restless anxiety*
AURUM METALLICUM	*Depression*
BORAX	*Dizziness*

CALCAREA CARBONICA	
CALCAREA PHOSPHORICA	
COCCULUS	*And lack of sleep*
KALIUM BROMATUM	*With continuous hand movements*
KALIUM PHOSPHORICUM	*Headache*
NATRUM CARBONICUM	*Headache, heavy head, dizziness*
NATRUM MURIATICUM	*Headache, dizziness*
NUX MOSCHATA	*Sleepiness at the slightest mental effort*
NUX VOMICA	*Insomnia, dizziness*
PHOSPHORICUM ACIDUM	*Heavy head, dizziness*
PHOSPHORUS	*Heavy head*
PICRICUM ACIDUM	*Frontal headache*
PULSATILLA	*Dizziness*
SELENIUM	
SEPIA	
SILICEA	*Fatigue*
ZINCUM METALLICUM	*With continuous restlessness of the feet*

INTERCOURSE (After)

CALCAREA CARBONICA	*Headache, burning pain in the urethra, shaking of lower limbs*
CHINA (CINCHONA)	
COBALTUM METALLICUM	*Lumbar pains*
KALIUM CARBONICUM	*Asthenia, headache, chills and shaking, weak sight with photophobia, insomnia*
KALIUM PHOSPHORICUM	
LYCOPODIUM	*Falling asleep*
NITRICUM ACIDUM	*Vaginal pruritus*
PHOSPHORICUM ACIDUM	
SELENIUM	
SEPIA	*Headache*
SILICEA	*Headache*
STAPHYSAGRIA	*Lumbar pain occurring during the night*
SULFUR (SULPHUR)	*Burning pain in the urethra*

ITCHING: *Pruritus*

ANACARDIUM ORIENTALE	
ARSENICUM ALBUM	*Itching until bleeding*
BERBERIS	
CROTON TIGLIUM	*Eczema with hypersensitivity to touch*
LEDUM PALUSTRE	
LYCOPODIUM	*Itching until bleeding*
MEZEREUM	
SULFUR (SULPHUR)	*Anal and limb pruritus*

JOLTS

ARNICA	*Muscle bruising, venous pain*
BELLADONNA	*Headache, mastodynia, facial neuralgia when walking quickly, when going down the stairs*

BERBERIS	*Hepatic or nephritic colic*
GLONOINUM	*Headache*
HAMAMELIS	*Venous pain*
HYPERICUM	*Neuralgic pain*
LAC CANINUM	*Mastodynia while going down the stairs, improved by wearing a bra*
LYCOPODIUM	*Heartburn*
NUX VOMICA	*Headache*
PHOSPHORICUM ACIDUM	*Headache*
PRUNUS SPINOSA	*Facial neuralgia*
SILICEA	*Headache if a step is missed*
SPIGELIA ANTHELMIA	*Headache on the left side, facial neuralgia*
TELLURIUM	*Sciatica*
THUYA (THUJA OCCIDENTALIS)	*Back pain*
VIBURNUM OPULUS	*Dysmenorrhea*

KNEES (In a kneeling position)

SEPIA	*Dizziness, palpitations*

LAND (Returning from sea)

BROMUM	*Sailors' asthma*

LAUGHING (While): *Cough*

CHINA (CINCHONA)
DROSERA
PHOSPHORUS
STANNUM METALLICUM

LAXATIVES: *Digestive disorders*

ALOE	*Diarrhea with sphincter insecurity*
HYDRASTIS	*Chronic constipation with no urges*
NUX VOMICA	*Constipation with false urges*

LEGS Dangling: *Venous pain*

BELLADONNA
PULSATILLA
SEPIA
VIPERA REDI

LIGHT Bright

ACONITUM	*Headache, photophobia due to sunlight*
ARGENTUM NITRICUM	*Headache, conjunctivitis*
ARSENICUM ALBUM	*Reflection off snow*
BELLADONNA	*Bright objects: conjunctivitis, headaches, convulsions*
CALCAREA CARBONICA	*Headache*

CHINA (CINCHONA)	*Photophobia due to sunlight*
CONIUM MACULATUM	*Photophobia due to artificial light*
EUPHRASIA	*Conjunctivitis*
GRAPHITES	*Photophobia due to sunlight*
MERCURIUS SOLUBILIS	*Conjunctivitis, ocular pain due to firelight or heat*
NUX VOMICA	*General sensorial hypersensitivity*
PHOSPHORUS	*General sensorial hypersensitivity*
SANGUINARIA CANADENSIS	*Migraine*
SEPIA	*Headache due to artificial light*
STRAMONIUM	*But improved by a soft, tempered light*
SULFUR (SULPHUR)	*Photophobia due to sunlight*

LOOKED AT (While being)

Irritability

ANTIMONIUM CRUDUM
CINA

Stuttering, shaking

ARGENTUM NITRICUM

LOOKING (While)

DOWNWARDS: *Dizziness*

ARGENTUM NITRICUM
OLEANDER
PHOSPHORUS
SPIGELIA ANTHELMIA
SULFUR (SULPHUR)

INTENSELY (An object)

NATRUM MURIATICUM	*Eye pain*
ONOSMODIUM	*Headache*
SPIGELIA ANTHELMIA	*Dizziness*

SIDEWAYS

CONIUM	*Dizziness*
KALMIA	*Eye pain*
SPIGELIA ANTHELMIA	*Dizziness*
TUBERCULINUM	*Eye pain*

UPWARDS: *Vertigo, dizziness*

ARGENTUM NITRICUM	*Looking up at tall buildings*
PHOSPHORUS	
PULSATILLA	

LYING DOWN, In bed

COUGH (With)

ARALIA RACEMOSA	*Asthma in early evening*

CONIUM — *And dizziness*
DROSERA — *Laryngeal tickling*
HYOSCYAMUS — *Improved when sitting: tickling in the nose and throat, nervous cough*
KALIUM BROMATUM — *During pregnancy; when the new moon rises*
MEPHITIS PUTORIUS — *Holding ones breath*
PULSATILLA — *Improved when sitting*
SENEGA — *Feeling of suffocation*
SEPIA — *Improved when sitting*

DIZZINESS (With)

CONIUM MACULATUM — *When moving ones head*

LEFT SIDE (On the)

BRYONIA — *Hepatic pain*
CACTUS — *Arrhythmia, dyspnea, palpitations*
CARDUUS MARIANUS — *Hepatic pain*
KALMIA LATIFOLIA — *Palpitations*
NAJA NAJA (NAJA TRIPUDIANS) *Palpitations with dyspnea*
PHOSPHORUS — *Except headache; diarrhea, chest pain, insomnia, palpitations, dry cough, dizziness*
SEPIA — *Sensation of "fullness" in the right upper abdomen*
SPIGELIA ANTHELMIA — *Palpitations*

RIGHT SIDE (On the)

ARGENTUM NITRICUM — *Palpitations, anxiety*
LILIUM TIGRINUM — *Palpitations, precordialgia*
LYCOPODIUM — *Hepatic pain*
MERCURIUS SOLUBILIS — *Hepatic pain, chest pain, cough*

MEAL

See also EATING (After)

KALIUM CARBONICUM — *Bloating while eating or drinking*
LYCOPODIUM — *Digestive disorders, facial erythrosis*
NUX MOSCHATA — *Bloating, sleepiness*
NUX VOMICA — *Far from a meal: 2 hours later*

MEAL (DELAYED MEAL)

ANACARDIUM ORIENTALE — *Generally far from meals, general improvement when eating*
CACTUS — *Migraine*
FLUORICUM ACIDUM — *Migraine*
IODUM — *Irritability*
KALIUM CARBONICUM — *Dizzy when hungry*
LYCOPODIUM — *Irritability, migraine*
PSORINUM — *Migraine*
SILICEA — *Migraine*

MEAT

See also **PORK, VEAL**

ALLIUM SATIVUM	*Dyspepsia for hearty meat eaters*
ARSENICUM ALBUM	*Rotten meat*
CAUSTICUM	*Nausea*
COLCHICUM	*Gout attack caused by foods rich in uric acid: giblets, etc.*
PULSATILLA	*Headache after eating fatty meat, pork*
STAPHYSAGRIA	*Digestive disorders*

MELON: *Diarrhea*

ARSENICUM ALBUM	*And watery fruit*
ZINGIBER	

MILK

AETHUSA CYNAPIUM	*Diarrhea and vomiting*
CALCAREA CARBONICA	*Dyspepsia, nausea*
CARBO VEGETABILIS	*Flatulence*
CHINA (CINCHONA)	*Flatulent colitis, nausea, slowed growth in children*
IODUM	*Diarrhea*
LAC DEFLORATUM	*Constipation and migraine*
MAGNESIA CARBONICA	*Diarrhea and vomiting*
MAGNESIA MURIATICA	*Constipation and gastralgia, nausea*
NATRUM CARBONICUM	*Abdominal flatulence, nausea*
NITRICUM ACIDUM	*Nausea*
NUX VOMICA	*Nausea*
PULSATILLA	*Diarrhea*
SEPIA	*Nausea*
SILICEA	*Diarrhea, slowed growth, vomiting breast milk*
SULFUR (SULPHUR)	*Nausea*

MOON (At the changes of the)

FULL MOON

CALCAREA CARBONICA	*Oxyuriasis*
CINA	*Highly typical general modality*
SABADILLA	*Pruritus located in: nose, ears, anus; spasmodic cough, abdominal colitis*
SULFUR (SULPHUR)	*Oxyuriasis*

FULL AND NEW MOON

CALCAREA CARBONICA	
CINA	*Pruritus: nose, anus; spasmodic cough, abdominal colitis, sleep disorders, bruxism*
SABADILLA	*Pruritus located in: nose, ears, anus; spasmodic cough, abdominal colitis*
SEPIA	
SILICEA	

NEW MOON

CUPRUM METALLICUM	*Convulsions*
KALIUM BROMATUM	*Sleepwalking, night frights*
LYCOPODIUM	
SABADILLA	
SEPIA	
SILICEA	*Highly typical general modality*

MOUNTAIN: *Acute Mountain Sickness (AMS)*

ARSENICUM ALBUM	
COCA	*General altitude-induced disorders*

MOVEMENTS

See also **PHYSICAL EFFORTS**

In general

AMMONIUM CARBONICUM	*Chronic cardiac or kidney insufficiency*
ARNICA	*In spite of the need to move around*
ARSENICUM IODATUM	*In spite of the urge to move around*
BELLADONNA	*General modality*
BRYONIA	*General modality: at the slightest movement; diarrhea, lumbar pain when turning over in bed*
COCCULUS	*Passive movement, sight of movement*
FERRUM METALLICUM	*Diarrhea*
GELSEMIUM	*General modality, except the heart-stopping sensation*
HYPERICUM	*Neuralgic pain*
IPECA (IPECAC)	*Nausea*
KALIUM CARBONICUM	*General modality*
LACHESIS MUTUS	*Aggravated dyspnea, arm movements, lower limb weakness*
MANGANUM	*General modality*
PHYTOLACCA	*In spite of the urge to move around; in flu syndrome*
PLUMBUM	*Neuralgic pain*
PSORINUM	
SANGUINARIA CANADENSIS	*Migraine*
SPIGELIA ANTHELMIA	*Neuralgia*
TABACUM	*Nausea*

BEGINNING of the movement (And improved by continuous movement)

CALCAREA FLUORICA
PULSATILLA
RADIUM BROMATUM
RHODODENDRON
RHUS TOXICODENDRON
TUBERCULINUM RESIDUUM

GOING DOWN (With downward movements)

BORAX	*Anxiety, nausea, dizziness*
CONIUM	*Dizziness*

FERRUM METALLICUM	*Dizziness*
GELSEMIUM	*Afraid of falling*
STANNUM METALLICUM	*Dyspnea while going down the stairs*

HEAD (During sudden head movements)

Torticollis

BRYONIA	
CAUSTICUM	
LACHNANTES	*Acute torticollis*

Dizziness while turning over in bed

BELLADONNA
BRYONIA
CONIUM

PASSIVE movement

See TRANSPORTATION

SLIGHTEST movement

ASCLEPIAS TUBEROSA	*Intercostal neuralgia*
BELLADONNA	*Pain*
BRYONIA	*General modality: pain, nausea, cough, dizziness*
DIGITALIS	*Heart-stopping sensation, arrhythmia*
ERIGERON	*Bleeding*
IPECA (IPECAC)	*Nausea*
NAJA NAJA (NAJA TRIPUDIANS)	*Precordialgia*
NUX VOMICA	*Headache, shivering*
RANUNCULUS BULBOSUS	*Intercostal neuralgia*
SABINA	*Menorrhagia*
SPIGELIA ANTHELMIA	*Precordialgia*
TRILLIUM PENDULUM	*Menorrhagia*

MUSIC (By classical)

AMBRA GRISEA	*Head congestion or cough*
GRAPHITES	*Crying*
NATRUM CARBONICUM	*Cries when listening to piano music*
NATRUM MURIATICUM	*Crying*
NATRUM SULFURICUM	*Crying*
THUYA (THUJA OCCIDENTALIS)	*Crying*
TARENTULA HISPANA	*With sweating*

NEW MOON

See MOON

NEWS (BAD NEWS)

See EMOTIONS

NIGHT

See TIMETABLE

NOISE

AURUM METALLICUM	
BELLADONNA	
BORAX	
CAPSICUM	*General sensorial hypersensitivity*
CAUSTICUM	*Afraid of noise*
CHINA (CINCHONA)	
COCCULUS	*Fits of anger, nausea, dizziness*
COFFEA TOSTA	*Limb pain, sensitivity to noise of footsteps*
GLONOINUM	
KALIUM CARBONICUM	*Which makes one jump*
KALIUM PHOSPHORICUM	
NATRUM CARBONICUM	*Hypersensitivity to music during menstruation*
NATRUM MURIATICUM	*Palpitations with any strange noise*
NATRUM SULFURICUM	
NITRICUM ACIDUM	
NUX VOMICA	*Irritability*
OPIUM	*Auditory hyperesthesia; insomnia with hyperacusis*
PHOSPHORICUM ACIDUM	*Headache*
PHOSPHORUS	*Sensorial hyperesthesia*
SANGUINARIA CANADENSIS	*Headache*
SILICEA	*Anxiety*
SULFUR (SULPHUR)	*Awakened by any noise: "cat nap"*
THERIDION	*With hypersensitivity to the slightest noise, nausea, dizziness*
ZINCUM METALLICUM	

ODORS

In general

AURUM METALLICUM	
CHINA (CINCHONA)	
COLCHICUM	*Medicine bearing this modality to the highest degree*
GRAPHITES	
IGNATIA	*Other people's odors, etc.*
LYCOPODIUM	
NUX VOMICA	*Fainting spell, syncope*
PHOSPHORUS	*Heightened sense of smell during headaches*
SEPIA	
SULFUR (SULPHUR)	

FLOWERS

GRAPHITES	
IGNATIA	
LAC CANINUM	
NUX VOMICA	*Dizziness*

PHOSPHORUS	*Dizziness*
SABADILLA	*Rhinitis*
SANGUINARIA CANADENSIS	*Migraine, rhinitis*

FOODS, COOKING

ARSENICUM ALBUM	*Nausea caused by smell of cooking and sight of food*
COCCULUS	*Nausea caused by smell of cooking*
COLCHICUM	*Cooking foods; eggs, fish*
DIGITALIS	
IPECA (IPECAC)	
SEPIA	*Nausea caused by smell of food*
STANNUM METALLICUM	*Nausea caused by smell of cooking*

GAS

PETROLEUM	*Motion sickness, smell of gas or exhaust pipes*

STRONG

PHOSPHORUS	*Cough*
SELENIUM	*Headaches*

SWEAT

SULFUR (SULPHUR)	*Nausea caused by ones own body's fetid sweat, due to lack of hygiene.*

TOBACCO (Smoke)

BROMUM	
CICUTA VIROSA	
COCCULUS	
IGNATIA	*Other people's smoke*
NUX VOMICA	

UNPLEASANT odors, odor of feces

SULFUR (SULPHUR)

ONIONS

LYCOPODIUM
THUYA (THUJA OCCIDENTALIS)

OVEREXERTION Intellectual, Mental

See **INTELLECTUAL EFFORTS**

OVEREXERTION Physical

See **PHYSICAL EFFORTS**

OVEREXERTION Visual

ARGENTUM NITRICUM	*Photophobia, eye redness*
BRYONIA	*Ocular pain*
DULCAMARA	*Eye numbness when reading*
GRAPHITES	*Dizziness*
MAGNESIA PHOSPHORICA	*Dizziness*

NATRUM MURIATICUM — *Often pricks a finger when sewing; dizziness*
NUX VOMICA — *Accommodation fatigue*
ONOSMODIUM — *Occipital headache, eye numbness*
PHOSPHORUS — *Dizziness*
PHYSOSTIGMA — *Blepharo-spasm, ocular pain, photophobia, accommodation disorders*
RADIUM BROMATUM — *Pain and red eyes*
RUTA GRAVEOLENS — *Pain or heat sensation on the eyeballs; excess work on computer screen.*
SILICEA — *Dizziness*

OVEREXERTION Vocal

See TALKING (While)

OVULATION (Inter-menstrual syndrome)

ACTAEA RACEMOSA (CIMICIFUGA) — *And general aggravation during menstruation*
AMBRA GRISEA — *And at the slightest emotion*
HAMAMELIS — *Inter-menstrual bleeding with dark blood flow*
SABINA — *Inter-menstrual bleeding, red blood flow mixed with black clots*
SECALE CORNUTUM — *Oozing watery bleeding between periods, black blood flow*

OYSTERS: *Digestive disorders*

ALOE
BROMUM — *Diarrhea*
LYCOPODIUM — *In spite of craving*

PARADOXICAL, Illogical

IGNATIA — *General modality*

PASTRY

See FAT

PERIODS (Before)

CALCAREA CARBONICA
CALCAREA PHOSPHORICA
CAUSTICUM — *Bad mood before and during menstruation*
CYCLAMEN
FOLLICULINUM
KALIUM CARBONICUM
LAC CANINUM
LACHESIS MUTUS
LYCOPODIUM
MAGNESIA CARBONICA — *Coryza, sore throat*

MUREX	
NATRUM MURIATICUM	
PHOSPHORUS	
PLATINA	
PULSATILLA	
SEPIA	*Lumbar pain with bearing-down sensation*
SULFUR (SULPHUR)	
VIBURNUM OPULUS	*Uterine pain, cramps, pelvic heaviness*
ZINCUM METALLICUM	

COLD SENSITIVITY, CHILLS

LYCOPODIUM
PULSATILLA
SILICEA

CONSTIPATION

GRAPHITES
KALIUM CARBONICUM
LACHESIS MUTUS
MAGNESIA CARBONICA
NATRUM MURIATICUM
SILICEA

CORYZA, PHARYNGITIS

GRAPHITES	*With cough and hoarseness*
MAGNESIA CARBONICA	

DIARRHEA

BOVISTA
LACHESIS MUTUS

HOARSENESS

GRAPHITES	*With cough and coryza*

IRRITABILITY

CAUSTICUM
NATRUM MURIATICUM
NUX VOMICA
SEPIA

MASTODYNIA

APIS	
BELLADONNA	*Pelvic heaviness, bearing down sensation*
BRYONIA	
CALCAREA CARBONICA	*Pain in armpits*
CONIUM	

FOLLICULINUM
HELONIAS DIOICA
LAC CANINUM
LACHESIS MUTUS
PHYTOLACCA
PULSATILLA

PRURITUS VULVAE

GRAPHITES
KALIUM CARBONICUM
LILIUM TIGRINUM
MERCURIUS SOLUBILIS
SULFUR (SULPHUR)

SADNESS

CAUSTICUM
MUREX
NATRUM MURIATICUM
PULSATILLA
SEPIA

PERIODS (During)

IN GENERAL

ACTAEA RACEMOSA (CIMICIFUGA)	*General modality, pain proportional to the flow*
ARGENTUM NITRICUM	*General modality: dysmenorrhea, palpitations, headaches, digestive troubles*
COCCULUS	
FERRUM METALLICUM	*Tinnitus*
GRAPHITES	
HYOSCYAMUS	
KALIUM CARBONICUM	
LAC CANINUM	*Sore throat*
MAGNESIA CARBONICA	
NUX VOMICA	
PLATINA	
PULSATILLA	
SEPIA	
SULFUR (SULPHUR)	
VERATRUM ALBUM	*Dysmenorrhea with diarrhea and cold sweating*

COLD SENSITIVITY

PULSATILLA	
SEPIA	
SILICEA	*Cold and damp feet*
SULFUR (SULPHUR)	

CONSTIPATION

GRAPHITES	
KALIUM CARBONICUM	*Cold-sensitive*
NATRUM MURIATICUM	
NUX VOMICA	*Nausea*
PLATINA	
SEPIA	
SILICEA	*Cold-sensitive*

CORYZA

AMMONIUM CARBONICUM	
GRAPHITES	*With cough*
LAC CANINUM	

DIARRHEA

BOVISTA
VERATRUM ALBUM

DRY MOUTH

NUX MOSCHATA

HOARSENESS

GRAPHITES	*And pruritus vulvae*

PRURITUS VULVAE

GRAPHITES	*And hoarseness*

SLEEPINESS

NUX MOSCHATA

TOOTHACHE

AMMONIUM CARBONICUM	
LACHESIS MUTUS	*When the flow diminishes*
SEPIA	
STAPHYSAGRIA	

PHYSICAL EFFORTS

ARNICA	*Pain in muscles, epistaxis, insomnia, acute urine retention*
ARSENICUM ALBUM	*Weakness, insomnia due to fatigue*
BROMUM	*Cough following physical exertion*
BRYONIA	*Facial neuralgia*
CACTUS	*Precordial constriction "like an iron hand"*

CALCAREA CARBONICA	*Headache*
CALCAREA PHOSPHORICA	*Fatigue with agitation and instability*
CAUSTICUM	*Painful limbs at the slightest effort, with sensation of tendons being too short*
COCCULUS	*Neck tiredness, trembling*
DIGITALIS	*Arrhythmia worsened by the slightest movement*
GELSEMIUM	
HEPAR SULFUR	*Cold sweating at the slightest physical or intellectual strain*
IODUM	*Tachycardia, effort dyspnea when climbing*
KALIUM CARBONICUM	*Cough*
KALIUM PHOSPHORICUM	
LACHESIS MUTUS	*Dyspnea*
LYCOPUS	*Cardiac erethism, tachycardia*
NAJA NAJA (NAJA TRIPUDIANS)	*Cardiac cough with laryngeal constriction*
NUX MOSCHATA	*Sleepiness*
PHOSPHORUS	*Right cardiac insufficiency*
RHUS TOXICODENDRON	*Headache, lumbar pain after trying to get up*
SELENIUM	*With a desire to stay in bed*
ZINCUM METALLICUM	*And mostly intellectual efforts*

PORK: *Digestive disorders*

ANTIMONIUM CRUDUM	
CARBO VEGETABILIS	
CYCLAMEN	
IPECA (IPECAC)	*Nausea*
PULSATILLA	*Indigestion, nausea*

POTATOES, STARCHES: *Flatulence, bloating*

ALUMINA
COLOCYNTHIS
NATRUM CARBONICUM

PREGNANCY (During)

ACTAEA RACEMOSA (CIMICIFUGA)	*Anxiety, fear of childbirth*
AESCULUS HIPPOCASTANUM	*Constipation, sacroiliac pain, hemorrhoids*
ARNICA	*Lumbar pain, painful movements of fetus, varicose veins*
ARSENICUM ALBUM	*Nausea, vomiting*
CALCAREA PHOSPHORICA	*Pubic symphysis pain*
CALADIUM	*Vaginal pruritus*
COLLINSONIA	*Hemorrhoids and constipation*
IGNATIA	*Anxiety, depression, fear of childbirth, nausea, vomiting*
IPECA (IPECAC)	*Nausea, vomiting*
KALIUM BROMATUM	*Cough*
KALIUM CARBONICUM	*Lumbar pain, nausea, vomiting*
LACHESIS MUTUS	*Hair loss*

LYCOPODIUM	*Hair loss*
MERCURIUS SOLUBILIS	*Nausea, heavy salivation, vomiting*
MUREX	*Painful pubic symphysis*
NATRUM CARBONICUM	*Sacroiliac pain*
NUX MOSCHATA	*Sleepiness*
NUX VOMICA	*Constipation, hemorrhoids, nausea*
PULSATILLA	*Varicose veins*
SEPIA	*Chloasma, depression, hemorrhoids, nausea, varicose veins, vomiting*

PRESENCE of a third party

See STRANGERS

PRESSURE (On)

EYEBALLS

EUPATORIUM PERFORATUM *Bruising sensation, flu syndrome*

LARYNX: *Cough*

CINA
RUMEX

LIVER

CHINA (CINCHONA)
CHELIDONIUM

SUBSTERNAL NOTCH

STICTA PULMONARIA *Cough*

PUBLIC (In)

See also COMPANY, CROWDS

Hyperventilation syndrome

MOSCHUS *Suffocating sensation*

Shyness

AMBRA GRISEA
GELSEMIUM *With trembling*
PULSATILLA
SILICEA

RAIN (Before the): *Joint pain*

NATRUM SULFURICUM *"Barometer" pain*

REST

PAIN

ASA FOETIDA *Painful bones*

CALCAREA FLUORICA	*Painful joints, varicose veins*
FERRUM METALLICUM	*Painful joints*
MEDORRHINUM	*Painful joints*
PULSATILLA	*Painful joints, varicose veins*
RHODODENDRON	*Painful joints, neuralgic pain*
RHUS TOXICODENDRON	*Painful joints*
RUTA GRAVEOLENS	*Painful joints*

VENOUS CIRCULATORY DISORDERS

HAMAMELIS
PULSATILLA
SEPIA
SILICEA
VIPERA REDI

SALT, Salty foods

ALUMINA	
MAGNESIA MURIATICA	
NATRUM MURIATICUM	*In excess*
PHOSPHORUS	*In excess*

SEA (At the seaside)

APIS	*Back from a sea trip*
ARSENICUM ALBUM	*Short stay at seaside: asthma, diarrhea*
LUESINUM (SYPHILINUM)	*Improvement when in the mountains*
MAGNESIA MURIATICA	*And salty foods*
NATRUM MURIATICUM	*Long stay: weight loss, asthma, eczema, herpes, depression*
NATRUM SULFURICUM	*Painful joints, respiratory disorders*
SEPIA	*Asthma, herpes*

SEASON

See **the relevant season**

SHALLOTS

LYCOPODIUM	*Flatulence*

SITTING

AMMONIUM MURIATICUM	*Sciatica*
BELLADONNA	*Headache congestion*
CHELIDONIUM	*Dizzy when sitting in bed*
COBALTUM METALLICUM	*Lumbar pain*
KALIUM BICHROMICUM	*Coccyx pain*
LAUROCERASUS	*Dyspnea when getting up from lying down*
LYCOPODIUM	*Sciatica*

SLEEP

See Chapter SLEEP

SLEEP (Lack of)

COCCULUS	*Dizziness*
NUX VOMICA	*Dizziness*
SELENIUM	
PHOSPHORUS	

SLEEPING (While)

See Chapter SLEEP

SMOKING (After)

See TOBACCO

SNOW MELTING

See SNOWY

SNOWY (Due to snowy weather)

CALCAREA PHOSPHORICA	*Joint pain, rhinopharyngitis during snow melting season*
CONIUM	*General*
SEPIA	*General*

SOLAR CYCLE (According to the)

See TIMETABLE

SOLITUDE: *Fear of being alone*

ACTAEA RACEMOSA (CIMICIFUGA)	
ARGENTUM NITRICUM	*With fear of dying*
ARSENICUM ALBUM	*Fear of dying, sadness*
CAUSTICUM	*At night*
GELSEMIUM	
HYOSCYAMUS	
KALIUM CARBONICUM	*With fear of dying*
KALIUM PHOSPHORICUM	
LYCOPODIUM	
PHOSPHORUS	*With fear of dying*
PULSATILLA	*Needing company*
SEPIA	*Meanwhile rejecting company*
STRAMONIUM	*At night*

SOUP: *Digestive disorders*

CALCAREA CARBONICA	*Sensation of stones in the stomach*
KALIUM CARBONICUM	*Bloating*

SPACES (CLOSED or EMPTY): *Mental disorders*

ACONITUM
ARGENTUM NITRICUM
CALCAREA CARBONICA
LACHESIS MUTUS
STRAMONIUM

SPICES (Strong spices, chilies, peppers): *Gastritis, hemorrhoids*

ALUMINA
CAPSICUM
NUX VOMICA

SPRING

ALLIUM CEPA	*Hay fever*
ARSENICUM IODATUM	*Pollen-induced asthma*
EUPHRASIA	*Allergic conjunctivitis*
GELSEMIUM	*Hay fever*
LACHESIS MUTUS	*Toothache, asthma, hay fever*
LOBELIA	*Pollen-induced asthma*
LYCOPODIUM	*Eczema, migraine, duodenal ulcer*
NATRUM SULFURICUM	*Dermatosis*
PSORINUM	*And in winter*
RHODODENDRON	*Joint pain*
RHUS TOXICODENDRON	*Joint pain*
SEPIA	*Circinate herpes*
SULFUR (SULPHUR)	

SPRING and FALL

LACHESIS MUTUS
LYCOPODIUM

STANDING still

AESCULUS HIPPOCASTANUM	*Hemorrhoid congestion*
COCCULUS	*Menstruation with abundant blood flow, dizziness*
FLUORICUM ACIDUM	*Headache, sensation of heavy legs*
LILIUM TIGRINUM	*Pelvic heaviness*
MANGANUM	*Asthenia*
MUREX	*Pubic symphysis pain*
NUX MOSCHATA	*Weakness of the lower limbs*
PALLADIUM	*Pelvic heaviness*
PULSATILLA	*Headache*
SEPIA	*Dyspnea, fainting spells, sensation of abdominal heaviness*
SULFUR (SULPHUR)	*Asthenia, hypoglycemic spells, lumbar pain*
TUBERCULINUM	*Asthenia*

STANDING UP (While)

BENT OVER (From a bent-over position): *Dizziness*

BELLADONNA
FERRUM METALLICUM

LYING DOWN (From a recumbent position): *Dizziness*

ACONITUM
GLONOINUM
PHOSPHORUS

SITTING (From a sitting position): *Lumbar pain*

SULFUR (SULPHUR)

STARCHES: *Digestive disorders*

ALUMINA	
BRYONIA	*Lentils, peas*
KALIUM CARBONICUM	
LYCOPODIUM	*Lentils, peas*
NATRUM SULFURICUM	

STAYING UP LATE (Often)

See **Chapter SLEEP**

STOMACH EMPTY (On an empty stomach)

ANACARDIUM ORIENTALE	*General modality*
ARSENICUM IODATUM	
IODUM	*General modality*
LACHESIS MUTUS	
PLATINA	*Noisy eructation*
SEPIA	*Nausea*

STORMY (Due to stormy weather): Before (and during) storms

IN GENERAL

BADIAGA
LUESINUM (SYPHILINUM)
MANGANUM
PETROLEUM
PSORINUM
RHODODENDRON

ANXIETY

NATRUM CARBONICUM	
PHOSPHORUS	*Anxiety, agitation, pain*

ASTHENIA

NATRUM CARBONICUM
TUBERCULINUM

EXCITEMENT

LACHESIS MUTUS	
RANUNCULUS BULBOSUS	*Sciatica*
RHODODENDRON	*Rheumatism and neuralgic pain, fears*
SPIGELIA ANTHELMIA	*Neuralgia*
STANNUM METALLICUM	*Neuralgia*
SULFUR (SULPHUR)	*Agitation*

HEADACHE

MELILOTUS OFFICINALIS

JOINT PAIN

CALCAREA PHOSPHORICA	
MEDORRHINUM	*Asthma, rheumatism*
NATRUM CARBONICUM	*Painful rheumatism, fear, asthenia*
NATRUM PHOSPHORICUM	*Gout*
RHODODENDRON	*Before storms*
TUBERCULINUM	*Asthenia, sensation of bone numbness before storms*

SHAKING

GELSEMIUM

VENOUS DISORDERS

SEPIA

STRANGERS (In the presence of)

AMBRA GRISEA	*Delayed urination or bowel movement*
BARYTA CARBONICA	*Goes to hide due to shyness*
NATRUM MURIATICUM	*Classically urination or bowel movement*

SUGAR, SWEETS

ARGENTUM NITRICUM	*Digestive disorders: eructation and flatulence, nausea, diarrhea; gastralgia*
GRAPHITES	*And aversion; nausea*
IPECA (IPECAC)	*Nausea*
KALIUM CARBONICUM	*Digestive disorders*
LYCOPODIUM	*Gastralgia*
MERCURIUS SOLUBILIS	*In spite of craving*
NATRUM CARBONICUM	*Toothache*
SULFUR (SULPHUR)	*In excess*

SUMMER

ANTIMONIUM CRUDUM	*Dermatosis, diarrhea*
BRYONIA	*Diarrhea*
CROTON TIGLIUM	*Dermatosis, diarrhea*
DULCAMARA	*Diarrhea after catching a cold*
FLUORICUM ACIDUM	*General state, venous disorders*
GRAPHITES	*Dermatosis*
GRATIOLA	*Diarrhea*
IODUM	*Weakness*
KALIUM BICHROMICUM	*Dermatosis, diarrhea*
MEZEREUM	*Dermatosis*
NATRUM CARBONICUM	*Dermatosis, orange-colored diarrhea, weakness, solar herpes*
NATRUM MURIATICUM	*Solar herpes*
PHOSPHORICUM ACIDUM	*Diarrhea after feeling cold, in summer*
PODOPHYLLUM	*Diarrhea*
SULFUR (SULPHUR)	*Heat intolerance*

SUN (Heat of the)

ACONITUM	*Sunstroke*
BELLADONNA	*Sunstroke*
BROMUM	
GELSEMIUM	*Sunstroke*
GLONOINUM	*Sunstroke*
HYPERICUM	*Benign summer light eruption (BSLE)*
IODUM	
LACHESIS MUTUS	*Sunstroke*
MURIATICUM ACIDUM	*Benign summer light eruption (BSLE)*
NATRUM CARBONICUM	*Asthenia, headache, dizziness*
NATRUM MURIATICUM	*Benign summer light eruption (BSLE), migraine*
SELENIUM	*Headache, neuralgia, headache above eyeballs*
VERATRUM VIRIDE	*Sunstroke*

SUPPRESSION of a discharge or an eruption

IN GENERAL (GENERAL MODALITY)

LACHESIS MUTUS	
SULFUR (SULPHUR)	*Following suppression of an eruption; sweaty feet*
ZINCUM METALLICUM	

EXANTHEMA OR SWEATING

CUPRUM METALLICUM	*Convulsions*
DULCAMARA	*Any disease if cooler weather suddenly stops ones sweating*
MEZEREUM	*Post-herpetic neuralgia*
OPIUM	*Convulsions*
SULFUR (SULPHUR)	*Convulsions*

ZINCUM METALLICUM	*Convulsions and nervous chronic diseases*

HEMORRHOIDS

NUX VOMICA

LACTATION

CYCLAMEN	*Dizziness occurring at the same time*

MENSTRUATION

CICUTA VIROSA	*Epilepsy*
LACHESIS MUTUS	*Secondary amenorrhea, menopause*
NATRUM MURIATICUM	*Depression*
PHOSPHORUS	*Epistaxis instead of menstruation*
PULSATILLA	*Asthma, burning desire to urinate, headache, uterine pain, lung inflammation, lumbar pain, dizziness*
SENECIO AUREUS	*Amenorrhea with vicariate disorders: cystalgia, diarrhea, hemorrhaging, leukorrhea, migraine, cough*

NASAL DISCHARGE: *Sinusitis*

BELLADONNA	
BRYONIA	
LACHESIS MUTUS	
MERCURIUS SOLUBILIS	
PULSATILLA	
STICTA PULMONARIA	*Stuffed nose with sensation of pressure at the base of the nose, frontal headache*

SWEATING OF THE FEET

BARYTA CARBONICA
MERCURIUS SOLUBILIS
SEPIA
SILICEA
SULFUR (SULPHUR)

SWALLOWING (While): *Dysphagia*

BELLADONNA	
LACHESIS MUTUS	*For liquids more than solids, with pain radiating towards the ears*
MERCURIUS CORROSIVUS	
MERCURIUS SOLUBILIS	
PHYTOLACCA	

SWEATING

IN GENERAL

CALCAREA CARBONICA	
CHINA (CINCHONA)	*And any fluid loss: digestive, blood, etc.*

FERRUM METALLICUM	*And any fluid loss: digestive, blood, etc.*
MANGANUM	*Pruritus*
MERCURIUS SOLUBILIS	*General signs, fever syndrome*
NUX VOMICA	*Nausea*
PHOSPHORICUM ACIDUM	*And any fluid loss besides diarrhea*
RHUS TOXICODENDRON	
SEPIA	
STAPHYSAGRIA	
SULFUR (SULPHUR)	

ACUTE FEVERISH AFFECTIONS

ARSENICUM ALBUM	*Tinnitus, vomiting*
CHAMOMILLA	
CHINA (CINCHONA)	
EUPATORIUM PERFOLIATUM	*For headaches only*
FERRUM PHOSPHORICUM	
HEPAR SULFUR	
MERCURIUS SOLUBILIS	
OPIUM	
PHOSPHORUS	*Profuse night sweating with weakness*
PULSATILLA	
RHUS TOXICODENDRON	
SULFUR (SULPHUR)	

TALKED (When being TALKED to): *Irritability*

ANTIMONIUM CRUDUM	
CHAMOMILLA	
NATRUM MURIATICUM	*In an introverted patient*
NUX VOMICA	*Anger when obliged to answer*

TALKING (While), SINGING, after...

See **also DESCRIBING ones symptoms**

CONVERSATION (By)

AMBRA GRISEA	
IGNATIA	
NATRUM MURIATICUM	
PULSATILLA	*Blushes whenever talked to*

COUGH

CHINA (CINCHONA)	*When talking or laughing*
DROSERA	*Emetic and hacking cough*
PHOSPHORUS	*Painful laryngeal irritation, dry cough when reading out loud*
RUMEX	
STANNUM METALLICUM	*Weak and empty sensation in chest; if talking, singing or laughing*

DYSPNEA after talking

LACHESIS MUTUS
NAJA NAJA (NAJA TRIPUDIANS) *With palpitations*
SPONGIA

HOARSENESS due to vocal burnout

ARNICA	
ARUM TRIPHYLLUM	*Bi-tonal voice*
CAUSTICUM	
RHUS TOXICODENDRON	

PALPITATIONS

NAJA NAJA (NAJA TRIPUDIANS)

WEAKNESS

ALUMINA
STANNUM METALLICUM
SULFUR (SULPHUR)

TEA

CHINA (CINCHONA)	*Flatulent colitis*
NATRUM MURIATICUM	*Dizziness*
SELENIUM	*Headache, digestive disorders*
SEPIA	*Dizziness*
THUYA (THUJA OCCIDENTALIS)	*Gastralgia, neuralgia, headache*

TEETH BRUSHING (While brushing ones teeth)

COCCUS CACTI	*And when rinsing ones mouth: whooping cough, vomiting*
NUX VOMICA	*Mostly in the morning*
SEPIA	

TEETHING (In times of)

AETHUSA CYNAPIUM	*Diarrhea*
CALCAREA PHOSPHORICA	*Diarrhea*
CHAMOMILLA	*General modality. Irritability and general hyperesthesia*
IPECA (IPECAC)	*With hypersalivation, rhinopharyngitis and cough*
KREOSOTUM	*Diarrhea*
MERCURIUS SOLUBILIS	*With hypersalivation, rhinopharyngitis and cough*
PHYTOLACCA	*Need to clench ones teeth*
PODOPHYLLUM	*Need to clench ones teeth, diarrhea*
RHEUM OFFICINALE	*Diarrhea*

TEMPERATURES (Extreme temperatures)

ACONITUM	*Following dry cold weather; or sunstroke*
ANTIMONIUM CRUDUM	*Due to radiating heat and by cold bath*
ARSENICUM IODATUM	*Cold-sensitive with craving for fresh air; due to hot wind*

BARYTA CARBONICA	*Body cold, with headache*
COLCHICUM	*Rheumatism of the limbs in hot weather and damp cold*
FLUORICUM ACIDUM	*General modality due to both hot and cold*
GRAPHITES	*Cold-sensitive with craving for fresh air; pruritus worsened by the heat of the bed*
LACHESIS MUTUS	*Worsened toothache; hot and cold drinks*
MEDORRHINUM	
MERCURIUS SOLUBILIS	*Cold and atmospheric heat; in general, due to local heat in all acute conditions; local cold in chronic conditions*
NATRUM CARBONICUM	*Cold, drafts, but also hot weather and sun*
NATRUM MURIATICUM	*Cold-sensitive due to tiredness caused by excess sun exposure and heat*
PHOSPHORUS	*Cough worsened by going from hot to cold, and inversely*
PLANTAGO	*Toothache*
RUMEX	*Cough worsened by going from hot to cold, and inversely*
SELENIUM	*Cold-sensitive, drafts, but also in hot weather*
SEPIA	*Damp cold and damp heat*

THANKS (After receiving)

LYCOPODIUM	*Cries*

THINKING (about) AILMENTS

ARSENICUM ALBUM	*Anxiety*
AURUM METALLICUM	*Depression*
BARYTA CARBONICA	*Intellectual deficiency*
CALCAREA PHOSPHORICA	*Anxiety*
CAUSTICUM	*Anxiety*
CHAMOMILLA	*Painful pressure on the temples*
GELSEMIUM	*Nervousness*
IGNATIA	
MEDORRHINUM	*Pruritus, mental disorders*
NATRUM MURIATICUM	*Depression*
SEPIA	*Nausea*

THUNDERSTORM (Sudden barometric changes)

See also **WIND**

ARSENICUM ALBUM	*"Heavy" feeling in chest*
BADIAGA	*Respiratory symptoms*
HYPERICUM	*Neuralgic pain*
NUX MOSCHATA	*General state*
RHODODENDRON	*Joint pain*

TIGHT clothes

BOVISTA

CALCAREA CARBONICA	
CARBO VEGETABILIS	
CENCHRIS	
COCCUS CACTI	
LACHESIS MUTUS	*On all levels*
LYCOPODIUM	*Abdomen*
NAJA NAJA (NAJA TRIPUDIANS)	*Neck*
NATRUM SULFURICUM	*Abdomen*
NUX VOMICA	

ABDOMEN (On the abdominal level)

APIS
ARGENTUM NITRICUM
CALCAREA CARBONICA
CARBO VEGETABILIS
CAUSTICUM
CHINA (CINCHONA)
CROTALUS HORRIDUS
GRAPHITES
LACHESIS MUTUS
LYCOPODIUM
NATRUM SULFURICUM
NUX VOMICA
SEPIA

NECK (On the neck level)

AMYLIUM NITROSUM
APIS
CENCHRIS
CROTALUS HORRIDUS
LACHESIS MUTUS
NAJA NAJA (NAJA TRIPUDIANS)
SEPIA

THORAX (On the chest level)

CAUSTICUM
CENCHRIS
LACHESIS MUTUS
NAJA NAJA (NAJA TRIPUDIANS)

TIMETABLE (According to)

DAY, HOUR BY HOUR

- *10 a.m.*

NATRUM MURIATICUM	*Need to snack, rhinitis, headache from 10 a.m. to 3 p.m.*

- 11 a.m.: need to snack

IGNATIA	*Not improved by eating*
PHOSPHORUS	
SULFUR (SULPHUR)	
ZINCUM METALLICUM	

- 3 p.m.

THUYA (THUJA OCCIDENTALIS)

- between 4 and 8 p.m.

CHELIDONIUM	*Pain in the upper right abdomen or at the tip of the right shoulder blade*
FAGOPYRUM	*Pruritus*
LYCOPODIUM	*General modality from 4 to 8 p.m.: with digestive, respiratory, infectious, urinary and painful afflictions; headache; crying*

DUSK: *Anxiety*

CAUSTICUM
LUESINUM (SYPHILINUM)
PHOSPHORUS
PULSATILLA

EVENING: *Hoarseness, coughing*

CARBO VEGETABILIS
PHOSPHORUS

MORNING, AFTER WAKING UP: *Diarrhea*

BRYONIA	*General with movements*
NATRUM SULFURICUM	
SULFUR (SULPHUR)	

MORNING

CALCAREA CARBONICA	*Hoarseness*
CAUSTICUM	*Hoarseness*
MANGANUM	*Hoarseness*
NATRUM MURIATICUM	*Bearing down*
NUX VOMICA	*Dry coryza at night with discharge in the morning, hoarseness*
PODOPHYLLUM	*Diarrhea*

NIGHT

IN GENERAL

AMMONIUM CARBONICUM	*Nose blocked with dry mucus*
AMMONIUM MURIATICUM	*Woken up by sneezing*
ARSENICUM ALBUM	*Night anxiety; gets up often; restless sleep after 3 a.m., aches, fever, earache*
AURUM METALLICUM	*Cardio-respiratory disorders, bone pain*

CAUSTICUM	*Restless agitation of the lower limbs*
CHAMOMILLA	*Aches, fever*
COFFEA TOSTA	*Aches*
DIGITALIS	*Night pollakiuria*
FERRUM METALLICUM	*Diarrhea*
KALIUM IODATUM	*Headache, sore bones, neuralgia*
LACHESIS MUTUS	*Generally worsened by sleeping*
LUESINUM (SYPHILINUM)	*From sunset to sunrise, pain*
LYCOPODIUM	*Nasal blockage*
MAGNESIA CARBONICA	*Neuralgia*
MERCURIUS SOLUBILIS	*Coryza, aches, epistaxis, fever, leukorrhea, facial neuralgia, earache*
MEZEREUM	*Neuralgia*
NITRICUM ACIDUM	*Violent coryza*
NUX VOMICA	*Nasal blockage*
PLUMBUM	*Neuralgia*
PULSATILLA	*Nasal blockage, earache, dry cough*
RHUS TOXICODENDRON	*Painful joints, fever*
ROBINIA	*Heartburn due to acid reflux*
SABAL SERRULATA	*Pollakiuria*

DEPENDING ON THE HOUR OF THE NIGHT

- 1st sleep: enuresis

CAUSTICUM
KREOSOTUM
SEPIA

- 9 p.m.

BRYONIA	*General modality*

- in the evening, until midnight

ARALIA RACEMOSA	*Asthma during the first part of the night*
CHAMOMILLA	
SPONGIA	*Laryngitis*

- between 11 p.m. and midnight

COCCUS CACTI	*Paroxysmal cough followed by abundant mucus, as well as in the morning when waking up*

- midnight

ACONITUM	*General modality: anxiety, fever, angina pectoris, cough, neuralgia, etc.*
SAMBUCCUS	*Laryngitis*

- between midnight and 3 a.m.

ARSENICUM ALBUM	*Asthma, anxiety, diarrhea, fever, palpitations, vomiting*

- between 1 and 3 a.m.: asthma

NATRUM MURIATICUM

- 2 a.m.

DROSERA	*Cough*

- between 2 and 4 a.m.

KALIUM ARSENICOSUM	*Asthma, pruritus*
KALIUM BICHROMICUM	*Pain, sinusitis, digestive disorders*
KALIUM CARBONICUM	*General modality*
KALIUM IODATUM	*General modality*

- 3 a.m.

AMMONIUM CARBONICUM	*Nasal blockage, dyspnea*
THUYA (THUJA OCCIDENTALIS)	*Rheumatic pain, asthma, digestive disorders, insomnia, facial neuralgia*

- between 3 and 4 a.m.

CAUSTICUM	*Cluster headaches, cough*
NUX VOMICA	*Insomnia until 6 a.m.*
SULFUR (SULPHUR)	*Insomnia*

- between 4 and 5 a.m.

NATRUM SULFURICUM	*Asthma, pain*

- 5 a.m.: diarrhea

PODOPHYLLUM	*And in the morning*
RUMEX CRISPUS	*Impelling diarrhea with need to get out of bed; often with coughing*
SULFUR (SULPHUR)	*Impelling diarrhea with need to get out of bed*
TUBERCULINUM	

BONES *(Painful sensation at night)*

ASA FOETIDA	
AURUM METALLICUM	
DROSERA	*Hip*
KALIUM BICHROMICUM	*Punctate, erratic*
KALIUM IODATUM	
LUESINUM (SYPHILINUM)	
MANGANUM	
MERCURIUS SOLUBILIS	
MEZEREUM	
NITRICUM ACIDUM	*Painful "splitting" sensation in the long bones*
PHYTOLACCA	

COUGH *during nighttime without waking*

CHAMOMILLA
LACHESIS MUTUS
VERBASCUM THAPSUS
TUBERCULINUM

PRURITUS *nighttime*

See **Chapter SENSATIONS**

SWEATING nighttime

ARSENICUM ALBUM	
CALCAREA CARBONICA	*Head, and mainly occiput*
HEPAR SULFUR	*With a sour odor, sometimes night and day without stopping*
KALIUM CARBONICUM	
LACHESIS MUTUS	
MERCURIUS SOLUBILIS	*With a highly characteristic general aggravation*

PHOSPHORICUM ACIDUM
PSORINUM — *Palms of the hands*
SEPIA — *Cold sweats*
SILICEA
SULFUR (SULPHUR) — *Profuse, with insomnia*
THUYA (THUJA OCCIDENTALIS)
TUBERCULINUM

SOLAR CYCLE: *Pain, Headache, Migraine*

GLONOINUM
KALIUM BICHROMICUM
KALMIA — *Pain in eyeballs*
NATRUM MURIATICUM
PHOSPHORUS
SANGUINARIA CANADENSIS
SPIGELIA ANTHELMIA
STANNUM METALLICUM

WAKING UP (In the morning), in bed

ALUMINA — *Mental confusion, sensation of fright*
AMBRA GRISEA — *Asthenia, mental confusion*
COCCUS CACTI — *Coughing, and between 11 p.m. and midnight*
GRINDELIA — *Choking when waking up and going to sleep*
LACHESIS MUTUS — *Angina pectoris, anxiety, asthenia, asthma, headache, palpitations, choking, coughing, dizziness*
LYCOPODIUM — *Headache, bad mood*
NAJA NAJA (NAJA TRIPUDIANS) — *Angina pectoris, palpitations*
NUX VOMICA — *Asthenia, headache, coryza with mucus during the day and dry at night, digestive disorders, cough*
PHOSPHORUS — *Headache, mental confusion, palpitations*
PULSATILLA — *Asthenia, mental confusion*
SAMBUCUS — *Facial sweat that stops if patient falls asleep again*
SEPIA — *Asthenia, headache, mental confusion, sweating*
SULFUR (SULPHUR) — *Asthenia, headache, mental confusion, profuse sweating*
TUBERCULINUM — *Asthenia, mental confusion*

BAD MOOD WHEN WAKING UP, IRRITABILITY

CINA
LYCOPODIUM — *And after a nap*
NATRUM SULFURICUM — *Improvement after abundant stools*
NUX VOMICA
TUBERCULINUM

DIARRHEA (WOKEN UP BY)

ALOE
PODOPHYLLUM
RUMEX — *At 5 a.m. mostly, with coughing*

SULFUR (SULPHUR)
TUBERCULINUM

NAUSEA

NUX VOMICA	
SEPIA	*Improved by breakfast*

TOBACCO (While smoking, second-hand smoking)

COCCULUS	*Nausea*
GELSEMIUM	*Dizziness*
HEPAR SULFUR	*Weakness, trembling*
IGNATIA	*Hiccups after smoking*
IPECA (IPECAC)	*Nausea*
NATRUM MURIATICUM	*Dizziness*
NUX VOMICA	*Nausea, dizziness*
SPIGELIA ANTHELMIA	*Neuralgia*
TABACUM	*Dizziness*

TOUCH Light, At the slightest touch

ACONITUM	*Larynx*
ACTAEA RACEMOSA (CIMICIFUGA)	*Spine*
ANTIMONIUM CRUDUM	*Toothache when touching the teeth with the tongue*
APIS	*General modality*
ARGENTUM METALLICUM	*Nasal cartilage*
ARGENTUM NITRICUM	*Neck*
ARNICA	*Bruising sensation, gout attack*
ASA FOETIDA	*Except painful colic; painful bones, ulcerations*
BELLADONNA	*General modality*
BERBERIS	*High lumbar area on the left, renal colic*
BRYONIA	*General modality, with improvement by strong pressure*
CANTHARIS	*Cutaneous hyperesthesia in the area of the afflicted organs: throat, abdomen, kidney, bladder*
CAPSICUM	*Mastoiditis*
CARBO VEGETABILIS	*Scalp: intolerance to wearing a hat*
CASTOR EQUI	*Tenderness in nipples when in contact with clothes*
CAUSTICUM	*Painful skin, burning sensation*
CENCHRIS	*Neck*
CHINA (CINCHONA)	*General modality*
CICUTA VIROSA	*Convulsions*
CINA	*Irritability*
COCCUS CACTI	*Nausea when touching the pharynx*
COLCHICUM	*Gout*
COLOCYNTHIS	*Facial neuralgia*
CROTALUS HORRIDUS	*Waist*
CROTON TIGLIUM	*Tenderness in nipples when in contact with clothes; rashes that are hypersensitive to touch*
CUPRUM METALLICUM	*Convulsions*
GRAPHITES	*Waist*

HAMAMELIS	*Varicose veins*
HEPAR SULFUR	*General modality*
HYDRASTIS	*Substernal notch, with coughing*
HYOSCYAMUS	
HYPERICUM	*Neuralgia*
KALIUM CARBONICUM	*Jumps at the slightest touch; very ticklish*
LAC CANINUM	*Mastodynia*
LACHESIS MUTUS	*General modality: cough worsened when the larynx is touched*
LYCOPODIUM	*Waist*
MAGNESIA CARBONICA	*Facial neuralgia, toothache*
NATRUM CARBONICUM	*Gastralgia when touching the stomach area*
NATRUM SULFURICUM	*Waist*
NUX VOMICA	*General modality*
MEDORRHINUM	*Joint pain*
MERCURIUS CORROSIVUS	*General modality*
MEZEREUM	*Pain in bones, facial neuralgia, toothache, pruritus*
MOSCHUS	*Hyperesthesia of the genital organs*
MUREX	*Hyperesthesia of the genital organs*
MURIATICUM ACIDUM	*Hemorrhoids*
NAJA NAJA (NAJA TRIPUDIANS)	*Neck*
NITRICUM ACIDUM	*General modality*
ORIGANUM	*Hyperesthesia of the genital organs*
PARIS QUADRIFOLIA	*Facial neuralgia*
PETROLEUM	*Eczema on nipples*
PHOSPHORUS	*Scalp, larynx, spine; very ticklish*
PLATINA	*Genital organs*
PRUNUS SPINOSA	*Neuralgia*
RANUNCULUS BULBOSUS	*Intercostal neuralgia*
RUMEX	*Substernal notch, with cough*
SEPIA	*Neck, with hot flashes*
SILICEA	*Neuralgia*
SOLIDAGO	*High lumbar area on the right*
SPONGIA	*Larynx*
STAPHYSAGRIA	*Hyperesthesia of genital organs*
TARENTULA HISPANA	*Of the spine with spasms, of the fingertips, of the genital organs*
TELLURIUM	*Vertebra C7 to T5 and lumbar spine*
TEREBINTHINA	*Abdomen, if infection*
THALLIUM ACETICUM	*Pain in lower limbs with intolerance to contact with the sheets*
VERBASCUM	*Facial neuralgia*
ZINCUM METALLICUM	*Neck and junction between thorax and lumbar area*

TRAIN

See **TRANSPORTATION**

TRANSPORTATION (Using means of): *Motion sickness*

BORAX — *Downwards motion: air pockets in planes*
CAUSTICUM
COCCULUS — *Motion sickness, headache, improved by hot, stuffy areas*
IGNATIA
PETROLEUM — *In a train when sitting facing backwards*
SEPIA — *Headache, nausea*
SILICEA — *Headache after the trip*
STAPHYSAGRIA
TABACUM — *Improved by fresh air, often in cars*

TRAVEL: *Constipation*

IGNATIA
LYCOPODIUM
PLATINA

TURNING OVER IN BED (While)

See MOVEMENT

UNDRESSED (After undressing or after taking off clothes): *Pruritus*

ARSENICUM ALBUM
KALIUM ARSENICOSUM — *Psoriasis-like rashes*
NATRUM SULFURICUM
RUMEX CRISPUS — *And coughing*
STAPHYSAGRIA
SULFUR (SULPHUR)
TUBERCULINUM

UNDRESSING: *Chills*

HEPAR SULFUR
NUX VOMICA — *Taking hands out from under the bed covers*
RHUS TOXICODENDRON
SILICEA
TUBERCULINUM — *Taking hands out from under the bed covers*

URINATION (After)

BLADDER PAIN

CANTHARIS
MERCURIUS CORROSIVUS

BURNING PAIN IN THE URETHRA

CANTHARIS
NATRUM CARBONICUM
NATRUM MURIATICUM

URINE IN SMALL QUANTITIES: *Painful joints*

BENZOICUM ACIDUM
BERBERIS

VACCINATIONS: *Diseases following vaccination*

MEDORRHINUM
SILICEA
SULFUR (SULPHUR)
THUYA (THUJA OCCIDENTALIS)
TUBERCULINUM
VAB — *BCG (tuberculosis vaccine)*

VEAL

KALIUM NITRICUM — *Diarrhea*

VEGETABLES: *Digestive troubles*

BRYONIA
HYDRASTIS
NATRUM SULFURICUM — *Raw vegetables*

VEGETABLES Raw: *Diarrhea*

BRYONIA — *Cold raw vegetables*
NATRUM SULFURICUM — *And starches*

VISUAL EFFORTS

See **OVEREXERTION Visual**

WAKING UP in the morning: *Diarrhea*

See **TIMETABLE**

WALKING FAST (While)

Dyspnea

ARSENICUM ALBUM
AURUM METALLICUM
KALIUM CARBONICUM
NATRUM MURIATICUM
PHOSPHORUS
PULSATILLA
SILICEA
SULFUR (SULPHUR)

Palpitations

AURUM MURIATICUM
IODUM
NATRUM MURIATICUM
PHOSPHORUS
SEPIA

WATER (By), WASHING, BATHS: *Skin disorders, pruritus*

CALCAREA CARBONICA	*Skin cracking*
CLEMATIS ERECTA	*Pruritic rashes*
DULCAMARA	*Pruritus and rash in contact with cold water: pruritus due to water*
GRAPHITES	*Sweating of the head after washing*
MEZEREUM	
NATRUM SULFURICUM	
PSORINUM	*Cold water*
RADIUM BROMATUM	
SEPIA	*Skin cracking*
SULFUR (SULPHUR)	*And aversion; toothaches, eruptions, skin cracking*

WET (After getting)

ALLIUM CEPA	*Diarrhea after getting feet wet*
ANTIMONIUM CRUDUM	*Applying wet cloths*
BELLADONNA	*Wet head*
CALCAREA CARBONICA	*Headache, toothache*
CAUSTICUM	*Paralysis*
DULCAMARA	*Cystitis, diarrhea, urinary incontinence, nasal blockage after getting feet wet*
PULSATILLA	*Wet feet; amenorrhea, dysmenorrhea*
RHUS TOXICODENDRON	*Drenched by sweat, amenorrhea, headache, diarrhea, chills*
SENECIO AUREUS	*Amenorrhea*
SILICEA	*Wet feet*
SULFUR (SULPHUR)	*Applying wet cloths*

WIND

The notions of northern or southern winds should not be taken into account. Depending on the region, the season or the weather situation, a northern wind can be hot or cold (anticyclone in winter), and a southern wind can be hot and dry, or mild and damp (onset of a storm).

In general: Intolerance to wind, generally

ARSENICUM ALBUM
CALCAREA PHOSPHORICA
CARBO VEGETABILIS
CHAMOMILLA
EUPHRASIA
HEPAR SULFUR
LYCOPODIUM
NUX VOMICA
PHOSPHORUS
PSORINUM

COLD (General modality)

ARSENICUM ALBUM
BELLADONNA
CHINA (CINCHONA)
HEPAR SULFUR
KALIUM CARBONICUM
MAGNESIA CARBONICA
PSORINUM
SEPIA
SILICEA

COLD AND DRY

ACONITUM	*Angina pectoris, fever, neuralgia, laryngitis*
CAUSTICUM	*Neurological and ENT symptoms*
HEPAR SULFUR	*Laryngitis*
NUX VOMICA	*ENT symptoms*
SPONGIA	*Laryngitis*

HOT

ARSENICUM IODATUM	*Asthma caused by pollens*
LACHESIS MUTUS	*General modality*
SULFUR IODATUM (SULPHUR IODATUM)	*General modality*

HOT AND HUMID

GELSEMIUM	*Infectious syndromes*
IPECA (IPECAC)	*Asthma*
KALIUM IODATUM	*ENT as well as respiratory syndromes*
RHODODENDRON	*Mostly sensitive to electrical atmospheric variations before a storm*

HUMIDITY: Generally most medicines of the sycotic reactive mode

AMMONIUM CARBONICUM	*Nasal blockage, lung congestion*
ARANEA DIADEMA	*Fever, cubital neuralgia*
ASCLEPIAS TUBEROSA	*Left intercostal neuralgia, pleurisy*
CALCAREA CARBONICA	*General aggravation modality due to damp cold*
DULCAMARA	*Breathing and osteo-articular symptoms*
MANGANUM METALLICUM	*ENT symptoms*
NATRUM SULFURICUM	*"Barometer" type of patient, very sensitive to hygrometry*
NUX MOSCHATA	*Headache, hoarseness*
PHYTOLACCA	*Osteo-articular symptoms*

RHODODENDRON	*Joint and neuralgic pain*
RHUS TOXICODENDRON	*Muscular-articular symptoms*
THUYA (THUJA OCCIDENTALIS)	*General aggravation modality due to all types of humidity*

WALKING AGAINST THE WIND, DYSPNEA

ARSENICUM ALBUM
BELLADONNA
NUX VOMICA
PHOSPHORUS
SEPIA

WINE

See ALCOHOL

WINTER

In general

AURUM METALLICUM	
HEPAR SULFUR	
PSORINUM	*And spring*

DEPRESSIVE DISORDERS

ARSENICUM ALBUM
AURUM METALLICUM
PSORINUM

SKIN DISORDERS

AGARICUS MUSCARIUS	*Chilblains*
ALUMINA	
ARSENICUM ALBUM	
CALCAREA CARBONICA	*Cracking on hands*
CISTUS CANADENSIS	
HEPAR SULFUR	
PETROLEUM	*Cracking on hands*
PSORINUM	
SEPIA	*Cracking on hands*
SILICEA	
SULFUR (SULPHUR)	

WOOL (By contact with): *Pruritus*

ARSENICUM ALBUM
PSORINUM
SULFUR (SULPHUR)

WRITING (While)

CAUSTICUM	*Trembling hands*
MAGNESIA PHOSPHORICA	*Writer's cramp*
MERCURIUS SOLUBILIS	*Trembling hands*
PLUMBUM METALLICUM	*Trembling hands*
SEPIA	*Sweating, dizziness*

IMPROVEMENT MODALITIES

ACIDITY (Drinks)

PTELEA	*Digestive disorders*
SANGUINARIA CANADENSIS	*Great thirst with craving for acidity in digestive and respiratory disorders*

APPLE

GUAIACUM	*Gastralgia*

BENT in two

COLOCYNTHIS	*Digestive, renal and gynecological pain, neuralgia*
GNAPHALIUM POLYCEPHALUM	*Sciatica*
MAGNESIA PHOSPHORICA	*Fleeting visceral and muscular pain, neuralgia*

BENT OVER backwards

DIOSCOREA	*Spasms, visceral pain*
ZINCUM METALLICUM	*Can only urinate when leaning backwards or sitting*

BENT OVER forwards

ASCLEPIAS TUBEROSA	*Chest pain*

BOWEL MOVEMENT

GAMBOGIA	*Urgent, sudden and painful diarrhea brings relief*
NATRUM SULFURICUM	*Abundant and watery stools*

CHANGING POSITIONS

ARSENICUM ALBUM	*Anxiety*
NATRUM SULFURICUM	*Painful joints*
RHUS TOXICODENDRON	*General modality, painful joints, neuralgia, pruritus and muscle aching are improved*
VALERIANA	*Sciatica*

COLD

IN GENERAL

ACTAEA RACEMOSA (CIMICIFUGA)	*Headaches*
AESCULUS HIPPOCASTANUM	*Circulatory affections*
ALLIUM CEPA	*Respiratory affections*
APIS	*Inflammatory and rheumatism aches, pruritus, edema, tonsillitis*

ARGENTUM NITRICUM	*Except gastralgia*
BELLIS PERENNIS	*Circulatory affections*
BRYONIA	*Except non-congestive headaches and painful joints*
FLUORICUM ACIDUM	*Circulatory affections*
GLONOINUM	
IODUM	*Respiratory affections*
KALIUM IODATUM	*Respiratory affections*
KALIUM SULFURICUM	*Respiratory affections*
LACHESIS MUTUS	*Circulatory affections*
PULSATILLA	*Circulatory affections*
SECALE	*Circulatory affections*
SULFUR (SULPHUR)	*Asthenia*

APPLICATIONS (COLD)

ACTAEA RACEMOSA (CIMICIFUGA)	*Headaches*
AESCULUS HIPPOCASTANUM	*Hemorrhoids*
ALOE	*Hemorrhoids*
ANGUSTURA	*Muscle aches*
APIS	*Pain in general, pruritus*
ARSENICUM ALBUM	*Headaches*
BRYONIA	*Migraines*
FLUORICUM ACIDUM	*Varicose veins, pruritus*
GUAIACUM	*Painful joints*
IODUM	
KALIUM ARSENICOSUM	*Pruritus*
KALIUM CARBONICUM	*Hemorrhoids*
LACHESIS MUTUS	*Hemorrhoids*
LEDUM PALUSTRE	*Painful joints, pruritus, trauma*
NUX VOMICA	*Hemorrhoids*
OPIUM	*Headaches*
PHOSPHORUS	*Headaches*
PSORINUM	*Pruritus, local modality contrasting with general aggravation to cold*
PULSATILLA	*Headaches, painful joints*
RADIUM BROMATUM	*Pruritus*
SULFUR (SULPHUR)	
TUBERCULINUM	*Pruritus, improved by cold water*

COLD DRINKS

APIS	*Pharyngitis*
BROMUM	*Coughing*
CAUSTICUM	*Gastralgia, coughing*
COCCUS CACTI	*Spasmodic cough improved by a little cold water*
CUPRUM METALLICUM	*Digestive spasms, hiccups, cough*
IPECA (IPECAC)	*Coughing*
LACHESIS MUTUS	*Pharyngitis, coughing*
PHOSPHORUS	*Gastralgia, coughing*
PHYTOLACCA	*Pharyngitis, coughing*

PULSATILLA	*Gastralgia*
TABACUM	*Coughing*

FRESH AIR

ACTAEA RACEMOSA (CIMICIFUGA)	*Headaches*
AMMONIUM CARBONICUM	*Respiratory disorders*
BROMUM	*Respiratory disorders improved by the seaside*
CARBO VEGETABILIS	*Respiratory disorders*
IODUM	*General symptoms*
NATRUM SULFURICUM	*Asthenia*
SEPIA	
SULFUR (SULPHUR)	*Asthenia*

FRESH AIR despite sensitivity to cold

ARSENICUM ALBUM	*Dyspnea*
GRAPHITES	
LYCOPODIUM	
NATRUM MURIATICUM	*Asthenia*
PULSATILLA	*Respiratory and circulatory disorders*
TUBERCULINUM	*Asthenia*

COMPANY

KALIUM PHOSPHORICUM	*Mental state*
PULSATILLA	*Mental state*
STRAMONIUM	*Night terrors*

CONSOLATION, SYMPATHY

PULSATILLA

CONSTIPATION (General state)

CALCAREA CARBONICA
MERCURIUS SOLUBILIS
PSORINUM

CROSSING legs when sitting

MUREX	*PMS pelvic congestion with sexual arousal*
SEPIA	*Pelvic "heaviness"*

DANCE

SEPIA	*Circulatory disorders and mental state, headaches*

DARKNESS

BELLADONNA
GLONOINUM
SEPIA

DAY BEFORE a pathological manifestation

PSORINUM	*Headaches, migraines; very reliable symptom pointing to the medicine*

DIARRHEA

ANTIMONIUM CRUDUM	*Headaches*
NATRUM SULFURICUM	*Depression*
PHOSPHORICUM ACIDUM	*Without affecting the general state*
PODOPHYLLUM PELTATUM	*Headaches*

DISCHARGE

EPISTAXIS

HAMAMELIS	*Epistaxis with black blood improves the headache*
LACHESIS MUTUS	*Headaches*
MELILOTUS OFFICINALIS	*Headaches*
ZINCUM METALLICUM	*Headaches*

PHYSIOLOGICAL OR PATHOLOGICAL

AESCULUS HIPPOCASTANUM	*Hemorrhoids, pain improved by flow of blood*
HAMAMELIS	*Headache with "heaviness" improved by black blood epistaxis*
LACHESIS MUTUS	*Very good general modality. Improvement can occur with menstruation, epistaxis, ENT discharge, bleeding, skin suppuration.*
MELILOTUS OFFICINALIS	*Headaches improved by epistaxis, periods, hemorrhaging, abundant urination*
NATRUM SULFURICUM	*Soft stools or diarrhea improve the local signs, the general state and the bad mood in morning*
SENECIO AUREUS	*Improved by the arrival of delayed or suppressed periods*
STICTA PULMONARIA	*Headaches improved by nasal discharge*
SULFUR (SULPHUR)	*Headaches, sweating*
ZINCUM METALLICUM	*Neurological disorders, headaches, dysmenorrhea improved by menstruation, sweating, expectoration, diarrhea, epistaxis*

DISTRACTION

IGNATIA	*Anxiety, stress*

DIURESIS Abundant

APIS	*Edema*
BENZOICUM ACIDUM	*Joint disorders*
BERBERIS	*Urinary disorders*
GELSEMIUM	*Headaches*
LYCOPODIUM	*Urogenital and digestive disorders*
SOLIDAGO	*Urinary disorders*

DRY weather

NATRUM SULFURICUM	*General modality, real improvement of all disorders by dry and hot weather*
RHUS TOXICODENDRON	*Mostly muscle and joint manifestations*
SILICEA	*General modality*
SULFUR (SULPHUR)	*Dry but temperate weather*

EATING (When)

ALUMINA	*Headaches*
ANACARDIUM ORIENTALE	*General modality, intellectual fatigue, headaches, digestive disorders*
GRAPHITES	*Gastralgia*
IGNATIA	*Nausea*
IODUM	*Irritability*
KALIUM PHOSPHORICUM	*Headaches*
LACHESIS MUTUS	*Migraine*
PETROLEUM	*General modality, gastralgia*
PHOSPHORUS	*Anxiety, gastralgia*
PSORINUM	*Asthenia, depression*
SEPIA	*Nausea improved after breakfast*

EMOTIONS Happy

KALIUM PHOSPHORICUM	*Mental state*

ERUCTATION

ANTIMONIUM CRUDUM	*Eructation that tastes like foods*
ARGENTUM NITRICUM	*Painful and noisy eructations that relieve gastric bloating*

EXPECTORATION (By): *Dyspnea*

ANTIMONIUM TARTARICUM	*Lung congestion*
BLATTA ORIENTALIS	*Asthma*
HEPAR SULFUR	*Improved by hard-to-expel expectoration*
SCILLA (SCILLA MARITIMA)	*Lung congestion*
ZINCUM METALLICUM	*Asthma, cough*

EYES Closed

PETROLEUM	*Dizziness, nausea*
TABACUM	*Dizziness, nausea*

EYES Open

ARGENTUM NITRICUM	*Dizziness*
THERIDION	*Dizziness, nausea, motion sickness when closing the eyes*

FANNED (While being)

CARBO VEGETABILIS	*Dyspnea*

FRICTION (By)

CROTON TIGLIUM	*Improvement of pruritus by soft friction*
FORMICA RUFA	*Arthritis*
MAGNESIA PHOSPHORICA	*Spasms*
MEDORRHINUM	
PALLADIUM	*Right ovary pain*
PHOSPHORUS	*Spinal reaction to massage*
PLUMBUM	*Colic*
PODOPHYLLUM	*Upper right abdomen*
RHUS TOXICODENDRON	*Painful joints*

GAS (Emission of)

ASA FOETIDA	
CARBO VEGETABILIS	
CHIONANTHUS VIRGINICA	*Peri-umbilical colic*
COLOCYNTHIS	
GRAPHITES	
HYDRASTIS	
LYCOPODIUM	
NATRUM SULFURICUM	
RAPHANUS	*Confined gases that are difficult to evacuate. Improves the start of post-surgery intestinal transit*
SANGUINARIA CANADENSIS	*Migraines*

GENUPECTORAL (Position)

EUPATORIUM PERFOLIATUM	*Coughing*
MEDORRHINUM	*Digestive disorders, coughing and asthma in children*
PAREIRA BRAVA	*Urination*

HEAT

In general

ARSENICUM ALBUM	*Heat in all its forms except for the congestive headaches and dyspnea*
CAUSTICUM	*Damp heat*
CHELIDONIUM	*Except headaches*
CHINA (CINCHONA)	*Neuralgia*
COLCHICUM	*Painful joints*
FERRUM METALLICUM	*Except head*
HEPAR SULFUR	*Coughing*
KALIUM BICHROMICUM	*Except pruritus*
MAGNESIA PHOSPHORICA	*Neuralgia*
NUX VOMICA	*Except nasal blockage and hemorrhoids*
PHOSPHORUS	*Except headaches and gastralgia*
PSORINUM	*Except pruritus*

RHUS TOXICODENDRON	*Pruritus, aching joints, cough*
SILICEA	*In all its forms; hot and dry weather, stuffy heat, wraps*

APPLICATIONS (Hot)

AESCULUS HIPPOCASTANUM	*Superficial pain*
ARSENICUM ALBUM	*Neuralgia, pruritus, burning pain*
BRYONIA	*Neuralgia*
CANTHARIS	*Skin, mucous membranes*
CLEMATIS ERECTA	*Dermatosis, pruritus*
COLOCYNTHIS	*Neuralgia, spasmodic pain*
HEPAR SULFUR	
KALIUM BICHROMICUM	*Headaches*
MAGNESIA PHOSPHORICA	*Neuralgia, spasmodic pain, better improvement than for COLOCYNTHIS*
MEZEREUM	*Neuralgia, burning pain*
MURIATICUM ACIDUM	*Hemorrhoids*
NUX VOMICA	*Headaches*
PSORINUM	*General modality*
RADIUM BROMATUM	*Painful rheumatism*
RHUS TOXICODENDRON	*Vesicles dermatosis, painful joints*
SILICEA	*All symptoms, general modality*
STRONTIUM CARBONICUM	*Congestive headaches*
URTICA URENS	*Pruritus*

CONFINED (Heat)

COCCULUS	*Motion sickness*
PSORINUM	
SILICEA	*Can withstand, whatever the symptoms, stuffy or radiating heat*

DAMP (Heat)

CAUSTICUM	*Laryngitis, painful joints*
HEPAR SULFUR	*Laryngitis*
MEDORRHINUM	
NUX VOMICA	

FOOD AND DRINKS (Hot)

ARSENICUM ALBUM	*Coughing and digestive disorders*
CHELIDONIUM	*Milk improves symptoms and hepato-biliary disorders*
GRAPHITES	*Digestive disorders*
HEPAR SULFUR	*Pharyngeal aching, coughing*
KREOSOTUM	*Ovary pain*
LYCOPODIUM	*Pharyngeal aching, dyspeptic disorders and coughing*
NUX VOMICA	*Coughing, digestive disorders, toothache*
RHUS TOXICODENDRON	*Coughing*
SABADILLA	*Pharyngeal aching, coughing*
SILICEA	*Coughing*
SPONGIA	*Coughing, laryngitis*

HUMIDITY

APPLICATIONS (Damp)

ASARUM EUROPAEUM	*Headaches and ocular pain*
CAUSTICUM	*ENT*
HEPAR SULFUR	*Damp and hot applications*
	Respiratory disorders, suppuration of the mucous membranes

DAMP and RAINY WEATHER

CAUSTICUM	*Contractures of the flexors, muscle stiffness*
HEPAR SULFUR	*ENT*
MEDORRHINUM	*Asthma, rheumatism*
NUX VOMICA	*ENT*

INHALING deeply

IGNATIA	*Context of dystonia*
LACHESIS MUTUS	*Pharyngeal constriction*

ITCHING

ARSENICUM ALBUM	*Pruritus*
ASA FOETIDA	*Skin ulceration*
GRAPHITES	*Pruritus*
LYCOPODIUM	*Pruritus*
MURIATICUM ACIDUM	*Pruritus*
PETROLEUM	*Pruritus*
PHOSPHORUS	*Pruritus*
PSORINUM	*Pruritus*
RADIUM BROMATUM	*Pruritus*
SULFUR (SULPHUR)	*Pruritus*

LEGS CROSSED while sitting: *Pelvic "heaviness"*

MUREX	*PMS pelvic congestion with sexual arousal*
SEPIA	*Pelvic "heaviness"*

LEGS (DANGLING LEGS)

CONIUM MACULATUM	*Neuralgia*

LEGS Elevated

HAMAMELIS	*Congestion*
PULSATILLA	*Inflammatory venous pain*
SEPIA	*Congestion*
VIPERA REDI	*Inflammatory venous pain*

LIGHT Soft

STRAMONIUM	*Night terrors*

LOOKING sideways (While) or while converging

OLEANDER *Dizziness*

LYING DOWN

ARGENTUM METALLICUM *Coughing*
EUPHRASIA *Coughing*
LAUROCERASUS *Cough of cardiac origin*
MANGANUM *General state, coughing*
SELENIUM *Asthenia*
VERATRUM ALBUM *Vasovagal syndrome*

ABDOMEN (On the)

ALOE *Abdominal pain*
CHIONANTHUS VIRGINICA *Hepatic colic*
CINA *Abdominal pain*
MEDORRHINUM *Asthma, coughing*
PODOPHYLLUM PELTATUM *Abdominal pain*

HEAD LOWERED

ARNICA *Traumatic shock*
LAUROCERASUS *Dizziness, coughing and suffocating dyspnea*

MENSTRUATION

MENSTRUATION (During)

This modality is common in most women suffering from PMS. It is of greater value if a precise symptom does improve or if physical and emotional well-being is largely noticeable.

LACHESIS MUTUS *Mood disorders, congestion, gynecological, circulatory and digestive disorders*
PULSATILLA *General state, circulatory disorders*
SENECIO AUREUS *Amenorrhea with substitutive symptoms: coughing, migraines, lumbar pain, cystalgia, vicariating bleeding*
SEPIA *Coated tongue becomes clean during menstruation*
ZINCUM METALLICUM *Neurological disorders, dysmenorrhea, ovary pain*

MENSTRUATION (After)

ACTAEA RACEMOSA (CIMICIFUGA)

MOUNTAIN

LUESINUM (SYPHILINUM) *General modality*

MOVEMENT

At the BEGINNING of the movement

RUTA GRAVEOLENS *No painful warming up*

CHANGING position

ARSENICUM ALBUM *Anxiety*
RHUS TOXICODENDRON *Painful joints*

CONTINUOUS

In acute pathology

ARNICA
KALIUM IODATUM
PULSATILLA
RHUS TOXICODENDRON *Sciatica*
THUYA (THUJA OCCIDENTALIS)

In chronic pathology (rheumatism)

MEDORRHINUM
NATRUM CARBONICUM
NATRUM SULFURICUM
RADIUM BROMATUM
SULFUR (SULPHUR)
THUYA (THUJA OCCIDENTALIS)
TUBERCULINUM RESIDUUM

HANDS and FINGERS

KALIUM BROMATUM *Anxiety*

OUTSIDE In spite of feeling cold

CARBO VEGETABILIS
GRAPHITES
PULSATILLA
SEPIA

PASSIVE (Rocked, strolled, carried)

CHAMOMILLA *Nervousness, tantrums*
NITRICUM ACIDUM *Mood improvement when going for a drive*

QUICK

ARSENICUM ALBUM *Anxiety*
RHUS TOXICODENDRON *Painful joints*
SEPIA *Physical exercise, sports, particularly dancing, improve pain, migraine and mental state*

SLOW

FERRUM METALLICUM	*Painful joints*
GELSEMIUM	*Cardiac erethism*
KALIUM PHOSPHORICUM	*Asthenia improved by slow walking*
LYCOPODIUM	*Digestive disorders and pain*
PULSATILLA	*Venous stasis*

MUSIC

TARENTULA HISPANA	*Classic but controversial, need to be cautious of this pathogenesis*

NAP

NUX VOMICA	*Short*
PHOSPHORUS	

NOISE

CHAMOMILLA	*Insomnia*
IGNATIA	*Insomnia*

OCCUPATIONS

HELONIAS DIOICA	*Patients always feel better when distracted from symptoms*
IGNATIA	*Distraction improves symptoms*
IODUM	*Agitation, anxiety*
KALIUM BROMATUM	*Depression*
SEPIA	*Mental state, migraines*

PHYSICAL EXERCISE (By)

FLUORICUM ACIDUM	*Intense. Circulation*
KALIUM IODATUM	*Joint aches*
RHUS TOXICODENDRON	*Rheumatism and tendinous aches*
SEPIA	*Intense. Venous circulatory troubles and mental state*

PRESSURE (Strong pressure on the painful spot)

ARGENTUM NITRICUM	*Headaches*
BRYONIA	*Reliable general modality but aggravation at the slightest touch*
CHINA (CINCHONA)	*Pain aggravated at the slightest touch, improved by strong pressure*
COLOCYNTHIS	*Cramping pains*
EQUISETUM HYEMALE	*Bladder pain*
GLONOINUM	*Headache with improvement by placing a cold wrap around the head*
KALIUM CARBONICUM	*Lumbar pain, hemorrhoids*

MAGNESIA PHOSPHORICA	*Visceral and muscular pain*
PALLADIUM	*Right ovary pain*
PHOSPHORUS	*Improvement when lying down on the right side but sensitivity to touch*
PULSATILLA	
RHUS TOXICODENDRON	*Lumbar pain*
RUTA GRAVEOLENS	*Lumbar pain*
SEPIA	*Lumbar pain*
TRILLIUM PENDULUM	*Pelvic pain*

REST

ANACARDIUM	*Asthenia*
ARNICA	*Asthenia but moves around in the bed because of the pain*
BRYONIA	*General modality*
CALCAREA PHOSPHORICA	*Asthenia*
CHINA (CINCHONA)	*Asthenia*
COLCHICUM	*Pain*
DIGITALIS	*Cardialgia*
GELSEMIUM	*Asthenia*
HYPERICUM	*Pain*
LATRODECTUS MACTANS	*Cardialgia*
MANGANUM METALLICUM	*Asthenia, coughing, general symptoms improved when going to bed*
MERCURIUS SOLUBILIS	*General modality*
NUX VOMICA	*Digestive symptoms*
PHOSPHORICUM ACIDUM	*Asthenia*
PHOSPHORUS	*Asthenia*
PSORINUM	*Asthenia*
SECALE CORNUTUM	*Intermittent limping*
SEPIA	*Digestive symptoms*
SILICEA	*Asthenia*

SEA (At)

BROMUM	*Sailors' asthma*

SEA (At the seaside)

BROMUM	*Laryngitis, asthma, coryza*
MEDORRHINUM	*General modality of the medicine, improvement of the atopic, rheumatic and mental disorders*
NATRUM MURIATICUM	*A short stay improves asthma, rhinitis, appetite; a long stay worsens this*

SITTING

ACONITUM	*Cephalic congestion*
GLONOINUM	*Cephalic congestion*

GNAPHALIUM POLYCEPHALUM	*Sciatica, neuralgia alternating with paresthesia*
HYOSCYAMUS	*Cough worsened when lying down, improved when sitting*
PULSATILLA	*Coughing*
SAMBUCUS	*Laryngeal dyspnea*
ZINCUM METALLICUM	*Urination*

SITTING, Bent forward, elbows on knees and head between hands

KALIUM CARBONICUM	*Cardiorespiratory, digestive disorders,*
NICCOLUM METALLICUM	*Coughing*

SLEEP

CARBO VEGETABILIS	*General state, digestive disorders*
NUX VOMICA	*Short nap*
PHOSPHORICUM ACIDUM	*Asthenia*
PHOSPHORUS	*Insomnia before midnight, improved after sleeping*
SEPIA	*Extended sleep, tries to fall asleep but feels tired in the morning*

SOLITUDE

BARYTA CARBONICA	*Shyness, apprehends contact with others or going out*
GELSEMIUM	*Apprehends talking or expressing an idea*
NATRUM MURIATICUM	*Depressed or "distant" subject*
SEPIA	*Sometimes since childhood*
STAPHYSAGRIA	*Following injustice or bottled-up anger*

SQUATTING

PAREIRA BRAVA	*Urination improved by squatting, during an attack of renal colic. Prostatism*

STANDING UP

CAUSTICUM	*Bowel movement; constipation*

STORM (After the)

RHODODENDRON	*Sensitive to electrical atmospheric variations; neuralgia and rheumatic pain aggravated before storms or thunderstorms disappear afterwards*

STRETCHING (While)

ANGUSTURA VERA	*Tendon and muscle aching in the extensors*
RADIUM BROMATUM	*Neuralgia, muscle and joint aches*
THUYA (THUJA OCCIDENTALIS)	*Neuralgia, muscle and joint aches*
ZINCUM METALLICUM	*Neuralgia, muscle and joint aches*

SUMMER

AURUM METALLICUM	*Depression*
CALCAREA PHOSPHORICA	*Painful joints*
PETROLEUM	*Dermatosis*
PSORINUM	*Everything (general modality)*

SWEATING

BRYONIA	*During fever*
CUPRUM METALLICUM	*During fever*
GELSEMIUM	*During fever*
LYCOPODIUM	*During fever, improved by generalized sweating mostly concentrated on the chest*
NATRUM MURIATICUM	*Headaches*
SULFUR (SULPHUR)	*Irritant acidic sweat improving the feverish state*
THUYA (THUJA OCCIDENTALIS)	*General modality*

TEETH GRINDING (While)

PHYTOLACCA	*Teething*
PRUNUS SPINOSA	*Neuralgia in teeth*

TIMETABLE

MORNING

CALCAREA CARBONICA	*After breakfast*
MERCURIUS	
PHOSPHORUS	

EVENING

LACHESIS MUTUS	*Great nighttime activity*
LYCOPODIUM	*After 8 p.m.*
MEDORRHINUM	*At nightfall*
TUBERCULINUM	

NIGHT

MEDORRHINUM

TRAVELING

TUBERCULINUM	*Likes traveling and differing activities*

URINATION Abundant

APIS	*Edemas*
BENZOICUM ACIDUM	*Joint disorders*
BERBERIS	*Urinary disorders*
GELSEMIUM	*Congestive headaches or ophthalmic migraines*

IGNATIA	*Spike-like migraine*
LITHIUM CARBONICUM	*Rheumatic pain*
LYCOPODIUM	*Urogenital and digestive disorders*
SILICEA	*Occipital or right occipital-frontal headache*
SOLIDAGO	*Urinary disorders*
STAPHYSAGRIA	*Post-urination burning sensation that stops when urinating again*

VOMITING

COCCUS CACTI	*Coughing improved by vomiting mucus*
NUX VOMICA	*Digestive symptoms, induced vomiting*
SANGUINARIA CANADENSIS	*Migraine*

PERIODICITIES, ALTERNATIONS, LATERALITY

These three concepts have been combined in a short chapter and should be studied carefully.

Periodicities are in fact rhythm modalities characterized by time periods of aggravation. Essentially these involve the influence of the solar cycle and lunar phases, as well as periodical aggravations at more or less fixed intervals, all empiric notions familiar to homeopaths and prefiguring or recalling those used in chronobiology. In earlier books, this topic was widely expounded on, from the onset of symptoms every day at the same time (the famous CEDRON, but also others) to the annual pathologies of certain medicines like PSORINUM (logical for ENT or spring allergy problems, but more interesting in winter-recurrence worsening), including symptoms occurring every two days, every three weeks, every six weeks, and so on. These concepts of duration seemed essentially bookish to us, with few or no practical applications; this is why we kept only headings that seemed reliable enough.

Alternations are also an interesting category, but are limited in number. They emanate from either a real pathological alternation within a pathogenesis like CROTON TIGLIUM where diarrhea and eczema can alternate, or from the ambivalence of certain medicines like NATRUM MURIATICUM denoted by dryness or hypersecretion of the mucous membranes, or from a mood description like alternating excitation and depression during a given day with ARSENICUM ALBUM. At any rate, alternations are only telltale signs, and a medicine should only be confirmed once all the symptoms of a patient are taken into account.

Laterality, also largely discussed in earlier books, can only be qualified as "preponderant". In fact people using LYCOPODIUM regularly as chronic treatment are more inclined, but not exclusively, to have their symptoms or morbid disorders (migraines, hepato-vesicular, circulatory or cutaneous problems) on the right side; a "general" right laterality is often mentioned. Likewise, a headache on the right side going from the occiput and settling above the right eye evokes SANGUINARIA CANADENSIS. In this case a "local" right laterality for this medicine is mentioned. Just as for periodicities and alternations, we have tried to keep only laterality found useful in practice, while bearing in mind that a lack of laterality, or sometimes even laterality contrary to the one corresponding to a patient's symptoms, should not rule out a medicine which is otherwise appropriate. Furthermore, so-called "crossed" symptoms (left shoulder/right hip, for example) have not been dealt with in this Memento, since clinical experience has shown that this "classical" and ancient notion is not entirely reliable.

PERIODICITIES

ANNUAL or SEASONAL

See also **SEASON** in chapter **AGGRAVATION MODALITIES**

PSORINUM

DAILY

ARSENICUM ALBUM	*At night between midnight and 3 a.m.*
GELSEMIUM	*Headache with aggravation at 10 a.m.*
KALIUM BICHROMICUM	*Headache always occurring at the same time*
LACHESIS MUTUS	*Aggravation when waking up and improvement in the evening*
LYCOPODIUM	*Aggravation when waking up: bad mood; aggravation between 4 and 8 p.m.*
NATRUM MURIATICUM	*Aggravation at 10 a.m. or from 9 to 11 a.m.: fever, rhinitis, migraine, asthenia, need to snack, depression*
SULFUR (SULPHUR)	*Aggravation at 11 a.m.: need to snack, asthenia*

SUNDAY or day of rest (Headache on)

IRIS VERSICOLOR
LYCOPODIUM
NUX VOMICA
SANGUINARIA CANADENSIS
SILICEA
SULFUR (SULPHUR)

ALTERNATIONS

CONGESTION of the head / ICE COLD sensation of the head

CALCAREA CARBONICA

CONTRARY MODALITIES (Of) : *Sometimes aggravated, sometimes improved*

IGNATIA
NATRUM MURIATICUM
PULSATILLA
SULFUR (SULPHUR)

CORYZA (DRY CORYZA) / CORYZA (FLOWING CORYZA)

NATRUM MURIATICUM
NUX VOMICA
PULSATILLA

CRIES / LAUGHS (Telltale sign:)

HYOSCYAMUS
IGNATIA
NUX MOSCHATA
PLATINA
PULSATILLA

CUTANEOUS (Of symptoms): *Eczema* or RESPIRATORY: *Asthma, spasmodic coryza*

ARSENICUM ALBUM
CROTON TIGLIUM
LYCOPODIUM
NATRUM MURIATICUM
PSORINUM
SEPIA
SULFUR (SULPHUR)

DIARRHEA / CONSTIPATION

ANTIMONIUM CRUDUM
CALCAREA CARBONICA
CHELIDONIUM
IGNATIA
NATRUM CARBONICUM
NATRUM SULFURICUM
NUX VOMICA
PODOPHYLLUM
SULFUR (SULPHUR)

DIARRHEA / ECZEMA

CROTON TIGLIUM
SULFUR (SULPHUR)

DRYNESS / HYPERSECRETION OF THE MUCOUS MEMBRANES

NATRUM MURIATICUM

DRYNESS OF THE SKIN / SWEATING

APIS
NATRUM CARBONICUM

ECZEMA / RHEUMATISM

SULFUR (SULPHUR)

EXCITEMENT / DEPRESSION

ARSENICUM ALBUM	*Over the course of the same day*
AURUM METALLICUM	*Excitement alternates with depression*
IGNATIA	
LACHESIS MUTUS	*Excited in the evening and depressed in the morning*
NATRUM MURIATICUM	
PHOSPHORUS	
SEPIA	

HEADACHE / DIARRHEA OR HEMORRHOIDS

ALOE
PODOPHYLLUM
SULFUR (SULPHUR)

HEMORRHOIDS / ECZEMA or PHARYNGITIS

AESCULUS HIPPOCASTANUM
SULFUR (SULPHUR)

HEMORRHOIDS / LUMBAGO

ALOE
NUX VOMICA
SULFUR (SULPHUR)

HUNGER / ANOREXIA

CINA
FERRUM METALLICUM
IGNATIA
LYCOPODIUM
NATRUM MURIATICUM

JOINTS (Of joint pain) / DIGESTIVE DISORDERS

DULCAMARA
KALIUM BICHROMICUM *And joint pain/Respiratory disorders*

JOINTS (Of joint pain) / HEADACHE

LYCOPODIUM

NUMBNESS of the hands: *alternating sides or alternating with the feet*

COCCULUS *Or stinging*

PAIN / NUMBNESS: *Sciatica*

GNAPHALIUM POLYCEPHALUM

PHYSICAL DISORDERS or MENTAL (Of)

ACTAEA RACEMOSA (CIMICIFUGA)
LILIUM TIGRINUM
PLATINA
VALERIANA

REDNESS / PALENESS of the face

ACONITUM
BELLADONNA
FERRUM METALLICUM
FERRUM PHOSPHORICUM
LAC CANINUM
PHOSPHORUS

RHEUMATISM / CARDIAC SYMPTOMS

KALMIA

URTICARIA / GOUT

LYCOPODIUM
SULFUR (SULPHUR) *Or asthma/gout*
URTICA URENS

LATERALITY

ALTERNATION OF LATERALITY

LAC CANINUM — *Neuralgia, migraine, mastodynia, tonsillitis, etc.*
SULFUR (SULPHUR) — *Tinnitus*

LEFT

ACONITUM
BROMUM
LACHESIS MUTUS
SEPIA — *Varicose veins, migraines, ptosis*

Headache

LACHESIS MUTUS
NICCOLUM METALLICUM
SEPIA

Intercostal pain

ACTAEA RACEMOSA (CIMICIFUGA) — *Submammary pain*
ASCLEPIAS TUBEROSA — *Laterosternal pain*
RANUNCULUS BULBOSUS

Left breast

ASTERIAS RUBENS — *Pain with axillary irradiation*

Left kidney

BERBERIS — *Renal lithiasis*

Left lung (Base of the)

NATRUM SULFURICUM
PHOSPHORUS

Left ovary

ARGENTUM METALLICUM
NAJA NAJA (NAJA TRIPUDIANS)

Left shoulder

FERRUM METALLICUM

Ptosis

SEPIA

Sciatica

COLOCYNTHIS
KALIUM BICHROMICUM

Tonsillitis

LACHESIS MUTUS	
SABADILLA	*Improved by heat*

SYMPTOMS PROGRESSING FROM THE LEFT SIDE TO THE RIGHT SIDE

LACHESIS MUTUS	*All symptoms, mainly ENT (tonsillitis) and gynecological*
NAJA NAJA (NAJA TRIPUDIANS)	*Ovary pain, headache, tonsillitis, rheumatic disorders*
SABADILLA	*Tonsillitis*

RIGHT

ARSENICUM ALBUM
BRYONIA
CHELIDONIUM
IODUM
LYCOPODIUM

Base of the right lung

BRYONIA
CHELIDONIUM
KALIUM CARBONICUM
LYCOPODIUM
MERCURIUS SOLUBILIS

Migraine on the right side

KALIUM BICHROMICUM
LYCOPODIUM
SANGUINARIA CANADENSIS

Right hip

NATRUM SULFURICUM

Right ovary

APIS
ARSENICUM ALBUM
CENCHRIS
LYCOPODIUM
PALLADIUM
PODOPHYLLUM

Right shoulder

CHELIDONIUM
FERRUM PHOSPHORICUM
IRIS VERSICOLOR
SANGUINARIA CANADENSIS

Right wrist

VIOLA ODORATA

SYMPTOMS PROGRESSING FROM THE RIGHT SIDE TO THE LEFT SIDE

APIS
LYCOPODIUM

SENSATIONS

DEFINITION

There is no consensus as to the definition of the word "sensation". In practice, a sensation is what patients feel but also the way they express this, using their own words, simply (elementary sensation) or elaborately (complex sensation, "as if..."). It can thus be said that a sensation is **the oral expression of what a patient feels.**

By definition, a sensation is a subjective symptom, meaning not observable by the physician (even though a sensation can have a real impact on patient behavior, an impact observable by others, such as an agitated state due to a sensation of anxiety, or an itch impelling patients to scratch).

CLASSIFICATION

There is no satisfactory **classification** of sensations; different authors sometimes list them with the mental state, other times with the sensory organs or even with the general symptoms. For us, the classification closest to clinical practice seems to be the following:

1. **Painful sensations**, elementary sensations that patients express easily. The pain range covers seven degrees: burning, stinging, sharp, throbbing, cramping, bruising and sensation of an open wound, with some "half tones" (drilling, piercing, etc.). Other terms are often misleading (digging, stabbing, lacerating pain, etc.).

2. **Sensorial perception disorders** corresponding to the 5 senses (sight, smell, taste, sound, touch) to which we must add:
- *thermal sensitivity disorders* (chills, hot and cold sensations),
- *changes in appetite and thirst,*
- *general tonicity* (sensation of overall weakness or well-being) *and awareness* (sleepiness or hyper-ideation).

Sensorial perception disorders occur in three different modes: *hyperesthesia* and *hypoesthesia* (modification of intensity), and *dysesthesia* (modification of the sensation's nature or distortion, illusions, hallucinations, etc.).

SEMIOLOGICAL VALUE

From a semiological point of view, somatic **pain** is considered to be a **general sign**, on the same level as mental symptoms* (including mental or moral pain), food cravings and aversions. Among non-painful sensations, general sensations are listed within general signs, along with such objective elements as perspiration or fever; and local sensations are listed with local signs.

---

* Some mental symptoms were voluntarily included with the sensations: sensation of imminent death, affective indifference, hypersensitivity to pain, and so on.

SENSATIONS

Sensations are usually of pathogenetic origin: as such they deserve to be taken at face value, with discernment and discrimination.

The search for sensations is a key element of homeopathic interviewing. However, it remains a delicate task for different reasons:

- sensations are rarely expressed in a clear and spontaneous way by patients, more so during a first consultation;
- on the contrary, self-observation generated from the consultation can lead patients to report artificial sensations that are of no real value.

To summarize, "ideal" patients, who can observe and talk about their general conditions in truthful and moderate terms, remain rare!

ABSENCE

BOWEL MOVEMENT (Of): *Constipation with urges*

ALUMINA	*Rectal inertia*
BRYONIA	*Dry stools as if burned*
HYDRASTIS	
LYCOPODIUM	*Common in children*
OPIUM	*Rectal inertia*

HUNGER (Of)

ARSENICUM ALBUM	
CHELIDONIUM	
CHINA (CINCHONA)	*Appetite comes back after the first bite*
COCCULUS	
COLCHICUM	*Nausea due to food odors*
FERRUM METALLICUM	
IPECA (IPECAC)	
LYCOPODIUM	*Quickly satiated*
MANGANUM	*Permanent impression of satiety*
NATRUM MURIATICUM	*Anorexia nervosa, or on the contrary thinness despite a good or even increased appetite*
PHOSPHORUS	*Sometimes anorexia nervosa*
PULSATILLA	
SEPIA	*Sometimes anorexia nervosa*
SILICEA	
SULFUR (SULPHUR)	*With thirst*

OLFACTION (Of)

AMMONIUM MURIATICUM	*Common; with a sensation of plugged nose in spite of clear, abundant and watery mucus.*
KALIUM BICHROMICUM	

KALIUM SULFURICUM	
NATRUM MURIATICUM	*During allergic rhinitis*
PULSATILLA	*Often associated with loss of taste*

With nasal polyposis

CALCAREA CARBONICA
FORMICA RUFA
SANGUINARIA CANADENSIS
SANGUINARINA NITRICA
TEUCRIUM MARUM

PAIN (Of)

OPIUM	*Doesn't feel any pain, in spite of the intensity of the general signs*
STRAMONIUM	*Except headache*

Chronic hoarseness without pain

CALCAREA CARBONICA

Diarrhea without pain

BERBERIS	
CHINA (CINCHONA)	*Exhausting, post-prandial, early. Often after eating fruit. Extensive bloating*
FERRUM METALLICUM	*Post-prandial, at night*
FORMICA RUFA	*In the morning, during a meal, or after breakfast*
PHOSPHORICUM ACIDUM	*Identical to CHINA (CINCHONA) in acute or chronic conditions*
PHOSPHORUS	*Abundant, discolored, with rice-like grains*
RICINUS	*Very abundant leading to dehydration*

Indolent varicose ulcer

FLUORICUM ACIDUM	*With pruritus*

SENSITIVITY (Of) Of the mucous membranes

CARBONEUM SULFURATUM	*And of the skin*
KALIUM BROMATUM	*Pharyngeal, urinary, genital*

SEXUAL DESIRE (Of)

In men

AGNUS CASTUS	*Impotence and diminished sexual desire*
ARGENTUM NITRICUM	
BARYTA CARBONICA	*Due to early senescence*
CONIUM	*Mostly impotence*
GRAPHITES	*Libido sometimes intact but impotent*
KALIUM CARBONICUM	*Sometimes the contrary, with great weakness after coitus*
IGNATIA	
LYCOPODIUM	*Impotence due to loss of confidence, then little sexual desire*
NATRUM MURIATICUM	*Mostly impotent*
ONOSMODIUM	

PHOSPHORICUM ACIDUM	*Psychasthenia*
SELENIUM	*Mostly impotent*
SEPIA	*For both genders, frequent disinterest in any sexual activity*
SULFUR (SULPHUR)	
In women	
BARYTA CARBONICA	
CAUSTICUM	
GRAPHITES	*Very low libido*
LYCOPODIUM	
NATRUM MURIATICUM	*Frequent vaginal dryness*
ONOSMODIUM	*Depression linked to absence of sexual desire*
PHOSPHORICUM ACIDUM	
SEPIA	

TASTE (Of) During coryza

BRYONIA	*Changed sense of taste*
KALIUM SULFURICUM	
NATRUM MURIATICUM	*Digestive disorders*
PULSATILLA	*Common symptom in digestive and ENT disorders*

THIRST (Of)

During fever	
APIS	*Except during chills*
GELSEMIUM	*Mostly difficulty with drinking rather than a real lack of thirst*
IPECA (IPECAC)	*Very little thirst*
PULSATILLA	
In chronic states	
MANGANUM	
NUX MOSCHATA	
PULSATILLA	*Exceptionally intense thirst*

URINATE (Of the urge to)

ARSENICUM ALBUM	
CAUSTICUM	*Urinary incontinence during efforts and when coughing*
HELLEBORUS	*Due to oliguria or anuria in all critical states*
OPIUM	
PHOSPHORUS	
STRAMONIUM	

URINATING (Of sensation when): *Unconscious urinating*

ARGENTUM NITRICUM
CAUSTICUM
MAGNESIA MURIATICA

ACROPARESTHESIA

See NUMBNESS OF THE EXTREMITIES

ACUTE PAIN

See also THROBBING (Pain)

Pain appearing suddenly and disappearing slowly

PULSATILLA

Pain appearing slowly and disappearing suddenly

ARGENTUM METALLICUM *Headaches*
PULSATILLA *Not frequently encountered*
SULFURICUM ACIDUM (SULPHURICUM ACIDUM)
For all pain

Pain appearing and disappearing slowly

ARGENTUM NITRICUM
LUESINUM (SYPHILINUM) *Pain in bones with aggravation at night*
PLATINA *Spasms and compressions*
STANNUM METALLICUM *Neuralgic facial pain*

Pain appearing and disappearing suddenly

BELLADONNA *Throbbing*
CARBONEUM SULFURATUM *Paroxysmal fleeting neuralgia*
COLOCYNTHIS
IGNATIA *Erratic and fleeting pain, without organic problems*
KALIUM BICHROMICUM *Erratic and punctate*
MAGNESIA PHOSPHORICA
NITRICUM ACIDUM *Stinging pain*
PHYTOLACCA *In the joints and bones, sudden, very erratic*
SULFURICUM ACIDUM (SULPHURICUM ACIDUM)

AGEUSIA

See ABSENCE of taste

AGITATION

BERBERIS *Of the left lumbar fossa*
MEDORRHINUM *Lumbar area*
TEREBINTHINA *Renal area*

ALIVE in the stomach (Having something)

CROCUS SATIVUS
CYCLAMEN
SABADILLA
SULFUR (SULPHUR)
THUYA (THUJA OCCIDENTALIS)

ANOREXIA

See ABSENCE of hunger

ANOSMIA

See ABSENCE of olfaction

ANXIETY felt in the pit of the stomach

DIGITALIS
IGNATIA
KALIUM CARBONICUM
MEZEREUM
STAPHYSAGRIA

APPREHENSION of being in public places, with diarrhea

ARGENTUM NITRICUM	*Agitated*
GELSEMIUM	*Trembling and inhibited*

AROUSAL Sexual

CALADIUM	*Increased libido but impotent*
CANTHARIS	*Painful tenesmus during urinary infections Priapism*
CASTOREUM	*In women, with spasmodic dysmenorrhea*
CONIUM	*With weakness*
HYOSCYAMUS	*Tendency to exhibitionism during delirious manifestations*
KALIUM BROMATUM	*Obsessional ideas*
LILIUM TIGRINUM	*Associated to pelvic heaviness, "bearing down"*
MOSCHUS	*Hysterical manifestations*
MUREX	*Associated with uterine congestion and ptosis*
ORIGANUM	*In women*
PHOSPHORUS	*Alternating with impotence*
PICRICUM ACIDUM	*Violent arousal with priapism*
PLATINA	*Painful genital hyperesthesia*
RANA BUFO (BUFO RANA)	*Uncontrolled sexual urge with debilitated mental state*
STAPHYSAGRIA	*Frequent frustrations*
STRAMONIUM	*Erotic delirium*
TARENTULA HISPANA	

BANDAGE Tight

See also TIGHTNESS

AFFECTED PARTS (On the)

ANACARDIUM ORIENTALE	*Calves, head, back*
STANNUM METALLICUM	*With sensation of weakness*

HEAD (On the)

ARGENTUM NITRICUM	*Improves headaches*
CARBO VEGETABILIS	
DIOSCOREA	
IODUM	*Pressure at the base of the nose*
NITRICUM ACIDUM	
PLATINA	*Numbness in the temples*
STICTA PULMONARIA	*Sensation of pressure at the base of the nose*

KNEES (On the)

ANACARDIUM ORIENTALE
AURUM METALLICUM

LIMBS (On the)

PICRICUM ACIDUM	*Legs*
PLATINA	

THROAT (On the)

CROTALUS HORRIDUS	*Prevents patients from speaking*
LACHESIS MUTUS	

BEARING DOWN

See **WEIGHT**

BED too hard

See also **STIFFNESS**

ARNICA	*Feverish state with adynamia*
BAPTISIA	*Stomach flu*
PYROGENIUM	*Infectious syndrome*
RHUS TOXICODENDRON	
RUTA GRAVEOLENS	
SILICEA	*With bruising in the lumbar area*

BLOATING Abdominal

GENERALIZED

CHINA (CINCHONA)	*Distended abdomen with rumbling. No relief from passing gas*
GRAPHITES	*With rumbling and pain*
KALIUM CARBONICUM	*Right after eating, even very scant meal*
NUX MOSCHATA	*Gastric and abdominal flatulence with sleepiness right after a meal*
PULSATILLA	*Often caused by an over-rich meal*

Sensations

LOWER PART OF THE ABDOMEN

LYCOPODIUM — *Passing gas*
SEPIA — *With sensation of emptiness or heaviness*

Of the right colon

NATRUM SULFURICUM

Of the left angle

LYCOPODIUM
MOMORDICA BALSAMINA

UPPER PART OF THE ABDOMEN

CALCAREA CARBONICA
CARBO VEGETABILIS — *Aggravated when lying down*

BLOCKAGE of food in the esophagus

ALUMINA

BLOOD ready to burst out of the nose, eyes or ears

MELILOTUS OFFICINALIS

BONES (Pain in the)

Aggravated at night

ASA FOETIDA — *Osteitis of the long bones*
AURUM METALLICUM — *Osteitis of the short bones, inflammatory rheumatism like ankylosing spondylitis*
DROSERA — *Hip, long bones and vertebras*
IODUM
KALIUM BICHROMICUM — *Punctate, erratic*
KALIUM IODATUM
LACHESIS MUTUS — *Tibia*
LEDUM PALUSTRE — *Pain rising from below; right hip and left shoulder; gout.*
LUESINUM (SYPHILINUM)
MANGANUM
MERCURIUS SOLUBILIS
MEZEREUM
NITRICUM ACIDUM — *Stinging pain, as from a thorn or splinter, in the long bones*
PHYTOLACCA
RHODODENDRON — *Aggravated by stormy weather; erratic*
STAPHYSAGRIA — *Lumbar pain, gout*

No precise time

CALCAREA PHOSPHORICA
EUPATORIUM PERFOLIATUM — *Aching, as if the bones were broken*

FLUORICUM ACIDUM
PHOSPHORICUM ACIDUM *As if the bones were being scraped*
PULSATILLA *Erratic*
RUTA GRAVEOLENS
SILICEA

BREAKS in bones

AGARICUS MUSCARIUS *Mainly of the spine, while bending down*
EUPATORIUM PERFORATUM *Mainly wrists*
HAMAMELIS *Lumbar area*
THUYA (THUJA OCCIDENTALIS) *As if they were going to break, as if they were made of glass*
TRILLIUM PENDULUM *Sensation of hip dislocation*

BRUISING

ACTAEA RACEMOSA (CIMICIFUGA) *Para-vertebral thoracic area*
ARNICA *Of all muscles*
BAPTISIA *During a fever*
BELLIS PERENNIS *Abdomen, pelvis, breasts*
BERBERIS *Lumbar area*
COCCULUS
COLCHICUM
DULCAMARA
ECHINACEA *Infectious syndrome*
EUPATORIUM PERFOLIATUM *Eyeballs, wrists, chest, calves; flu syndrome*
FORMICA RUFA *Gout*
GELSEMIUM *Flu syndrome*
HAMAMELIS *Hemorrhoids, legs*
LEDUM PALUSTRE
LITHIUM CARBONICUM
MANGANUM
MEDORRHINUM *Lumbar area*
NATRUM SULFURICUM *Of the thorax: must compress the chest to cough*
NUX VOMICA *Head, back, lumbar area*
PHOSPHORICUM ACIDUM
PHYTOLACCA *With need to move around, without improvement*
PYROGENIUM
RADIUM BROMATUM
RHUS TOXICODENDRON *Which improves when moving, changing position*
RUTA GRAVEOLENS
TERBINTHINA *Renal area*
TUBERCULINUM *Before a storm*

Eyeballs (Of the)

BRYONIA *At the slightest touch*
EUPATORIUM PERFOLIATUM *Flu syndrome*

GELSEMIUM	*Flu syndrome*
KALMIA	*Facial neuralgia*
ONOSMODIUM	*Eye strain*
PHYSOSTIGMA	*Eye strain*
SYMPHYTUM	*Post traumatic*

BURNING PAIN

IN ACUTE DISEASE

ACONITUM	*Palms of the hands*
ALLIUM CEPA	*Nose*
APIS	*And stinging*
ARSENICUM ALBUM	*Intense like hot coals, for mucous membranes, skin and neuralgia*
ARUM TRIPHYLLUM	*Mouth*
BELLADONNA	*Skin, mucous membranes*
BERBERIS	*Urinary tract*
CANTHARIS	*Burning sensation of the skin, digestive and urinary tracts*
CAPSICUM	*Pepper-like burning, urinary and digestive tracks, ENT area*
CARBO VEGETABILIS	*Skin lesions and excretions, digestive, respiratory and circulatory tracts*
CAUSTICUM	*Skin, mucous membranes*
EUPHRASIA	*Eyes*
KALIUM BICHROMICUM	*Respiratory, digestive tracts*
KALIUM IODATUM	*Sinuses*
LEDUM PALUSTRE	*Joints*
MERCURIUS CORROSIVUS	*ENT, digestive, urinary and genital mucous membranes*
MERCURIUS SOLUBILIS	*Urinary and genital mucous membranes. Pain less intense than for the previous one*
MEZEREUM	*Nasal bones, periosteal inflammation of the long bones, mouth and pharynx*
PHOSPHORUS	*Internal and cutaneous burning. Fever with burning palms*
RATANHIA	*Anus*
RHUS TOXICODENDRON	
SANGUINARIA CANADENSIS	*Nasal and pharyngeal mucous membranes*
TARENTULA CUBENSIS	*And stinging, intense, acute inflammation of the skin*
TEREBINTHINA	*Urinary mucous membranes*

IN CHRONIC DISEASE

In general

ARSENICUM ALBUM	*Improved by heat, whatever the pathology*
CAUSTICUM	*Burning and numbness of the skin and mucous membranes*
GRAPHITES	
HYDRASTIS	*Digestive and respiratory mucous membranes*
IRIS VERSICOLOR	*The entire digestive tract*
KALIUM CARBONICUM	*Pain mostly throbbing, pulsating*

KREOSOTUM	*Gynecological mainly*
MEDORRHINUM	*Urinary and genital mucous membranes, skin in very localized areas*
NATRUM MURIATICUM	*Of the mucous membranes with alternation between dryness and catarrh*
NITRICUM ACIDUM	*Diarrhea and leukorrhea*
PHOSPHORUS	
RADIUM BROMATUM	*Skin and pruritus*
ROBINIA	*Upper part of the digestive track which differentiates it from IRIS VERSICOLOR*
SECALE CORNUTUM	*Like hot coals, improved by cold. This contrasts with the objective coldness of the affected areas*
SULFUR (SULPHUR)	

WITH PREFERRED LOCATIONS

BONES (Burning of the) nasal

KALIUM IODATUM

FEET (Burning of the)

GRAPHITES	
LACHESIS MUTUS	
MEDORRHINUM	
SULFUR (SULPHUR)	*Mainly at night*

GENITAL / URINARY (Burning of the mucous membranes)

APIS	
ARSENICUM ALBUM	
CANTHARIS	*Before, during and after urinating*
CAPSICUM	*As from pepper*
CAUSTICUM	
COPAIVA	*Before, during and after urinating*
KALIUM CARBONICUM	*Urethral*
KREOSOTUM	*With excoriation and bleeding*
MEDORRHINUM	
MERCURIUS CORROSIVUS	*With bladder tenesmus*
MERCURIUS SOLUBILIS	
NITRICUM ACIDUM	
POPULUS TREMULA	
PRUNUS SPINOSA	*Urethral pain when urinating, moving from the tip to the base of the penis*
STAPHYSAGRIA	*Urethral burn between urinations*
SULFUR (SULPHUR)	
TEREBINTHINA	*With bladder tenesmus, flow of black blood*

***INTERNAL* burning with external cold**

ARSENICUM ALBUM	
CARBO VEGETABILIS	
SECALE CORNUTUM	
VERATRUM ALBUM	*Contrasting with the cold skin and cold sweating*

***LUMBAR FOSSA* (Burning of)**

BERBERIS	*Left*
SARSAPARILLA	*Right*

***PALMS* (Burning of the) of the hands**

FLUORICUM ACIDUM	
LEDUM PALUSTRE	*Joints*
MEDORRHINUM	
PETROLEUM	
PHOSPHORUS	*With fever*
SANGUINARIA CANADENSIS	*And of feet, with fever*
SULFUR (SULPHUR)	

***SHOULDER BLADES* (Burning between the)**

ARSENICUM ALBUM
KALIUM BICHROMICUM
LYCOPODIUM
PHOSPHORUS
SULFUR (SULPHUR)

***SOLES* (Burning of the) of the feet**

CALCAREA FLUORICA	
FLUORICUM ACIDUM	
LACHESIS MUTUS	
LEDUM PALUSTRE	
LILIUM TIGRINUM	
MANGANUM	*With a sensation of dryness*
MEDORRHINUM	
PETROLEUM	
PSORINUM	*In spite of being cold-sensitive. Fetid sweat*
SANGUINARIA CANADENSIS	*With fever*
SULFUR (SULPHUR)	
SULFUR IODATUM (SULPHUR IODATUM)	

***SPINE* (Burning along the)**

ARSENICUM ALBUM	
LACHESIS MUTUS	
LYCOPODIUM	
MEDORRHINUM	
PHOSPHORUS	
SECALE CORNUTUM	
ZINCUM METALLICUM	*While sitting down*

***STOMACH* burns**

IRIS VERSICOLOR
ROBINIA

Improved by hot drinks

ARGENTUM NITRICUM
ARSENICUM ALBUM
CAUSTICUM

GRAPHITES
LYCOPODIUM
Improved by cold drinks
PHOSPHORUS

VERTEX (Burning of the)
GRAPHITES
LACHESIS MUTUS
SULFUR (SULPHUR) — *Hot head and feet*

BURSTING SENSATION

EYEBALLS (Of the)

PRUNUS SPINOSA — *Right*

HEAD (Of the) By coughing

BRYONIA
RUMEX

VEINS (Of the)

GRAPHITES
HAMAMELIS
VIPERA REDI — *Dilated and hard veins, aggravated by dangling arms or legs*

BUZZING in the ears

CAUSTICUM — *With hypoacusis*
CHENOPODIUM ANTHELMINTICUM — *Tinnitus, like cannon fire*
CHINA (CINCHONA) — *With auditive hypoacusis or hyperesthesia; sounds seem far off*
CHININUM SULFURICUM — *Similar to the last one, with dizziness. Circulatory or iatrogenic origin.*
FERRUM METALLICUM — *With dizziness*
GRAPHITES — *With hypoacusis, improved in the middle of the noise*
IGNATIA — *Improved when listening to music*
KALIUM CARBONICUM
KALIUM MURIATICUM — *Eustachian tube catarrh with tinnitus when swallowing*
KALIUM SULFURICUM — *With eustachian tube catarrh*
LACHESIS MUTUS — *Improved during menstruation*
LYCOPODIUM — *Following an ear infection*
NUX VOMICA — *Intolerance to the slightest noise*
PETROLEUM — *During dizziness. Intolerance to conversation*
PHOSPHORICUM ACIDUM
SALICYLICUM ACIDUM — *With rotational dizziness and hypoacusis*
SULFUR (SULPHUR)

CHILLS

In general

ACONITUM
ACTAEA RACEMOSA (CIMICIFUGA) — *Chills all over the body*
CAMPHORA — *Has the sensation of being cold all over, but cannot stand being covered up*
EUPATORIUM PERFOLIATUM — *Beginning in the lower back*
GELSEMIUM — *Along the back*
NUX VOMICA
PHOSPHORUS
PULSATILLA — *With a need for fresh air*
RHUS TOXICODENDRON

AIR (Needing some fresh)

PULSATILLA

BOWEL MOVEMENT (Before)

MERCURIUS SOLUBILIS

BOWEL MOVEMENT (After)

CANTHARIS
MERCURIUS SOLUBILIS

GOOSE BUMPS

MERCURIUS SOLUBILIS

PAIN (With)

CYCLAMEN
MEZEREUM
PULSATILLA

UNCOVERED (When): *Fever*

ACONITUM
HEPAR SULFUR
NUX VOMICA
RHUS TOXICODENDRON

CHOKING

See also **LACK OF AIR**

DAY (During the)

CUPRUM METALLICUM

ETHYL SULFUR DICHLORATUM	*Severe asthma, acute lung edema*
MEPHITIS PUTORIUS	*After coughing hard*
MOSCHUS	*Sometimes with chest pain*
NAJA NAJA (TRIPUDIANS)	*Angina pectoris*

GOING TO SLEEP (When)

AMMONIUM CARBONICUM
ARALIA RACEMOSA
CENCHRIS
DIGITALIS
GRINDELIA
LACHESIS MUTUS
NAJA NAJA (TRIPUDIANS)
OPIUM

IMPROVED WHEN LYING DOWN WITH HEAD LOWERED

LAUROCERASUS

CLAMP (IRON CLAMP)

See TIGHTNESS

CLAWS

See CRUSHING PAIN

CLINCHING of teeth: *Teething*

PHYTOLACCA
PODOPHYLLUM

COCCYX too long

KALIUM BICHROMICUM

COLD

GENERALIZED (Cold)

ARSENICUM ALBUM	
CALCAREA CARBONICA	
CAMPHORA	*Can be observed objectively. Feels like ice, to the touch*
DULCAMARA	
PSORINUM	
SILICEA	
TABACUM	
VERATRUM ALBUM	

LOCALIZED (Cold)

AGARICUS MUSCARIUS	*Chilblains*

AMBRA GRISEA	*Extremities*
BERBERIS	*Right temple, outside of the thighs, male genital organs*
CALCAREA CARBONICA	*Head, feet and legs: "as if wearing wet stockings"*
CAPSICUM	*Affected areas*
CARBO VEGETABILIS	
CONIUM	*Gas and stools*
DULCAMARA	*With pain*
GRAPHITES	*Occipital area, knees, feet*
NITRICUM ACIDUM	*Cold soles of the feet, cold urine during urination*
PETROLEUM	*Heart, abdomen, between the shoulders*
SEPIA	*Vertex, between the shoulders, feet*
SILICEA	*Head, affected areas*
TUBERCULINUM	*Back, like wet clothes*
VERATRUM ALBUM	*Head, mouth like after eating mints*

AFFECTED AREAS (Cold)

KALIUM CARBONICUM
SILICEA
TUBERCULINUM

AIR (With a need for)

ARSENICUM ALBUM
CARBO VEGETABILIS

AIR INHALED (Cold)

BROMUM
CAMPHORA
CORALLIUM RUBRUM

BREASTS (Cold) And nipples

MEDORRHINUM

EXTERNAL (Cold) In spite of a sensation of internal burning

ARSENICUM ALBUM
CARBO VEGETABILIS
SECALE CORNUTUM
VERATRUM ALBUM

EXTREMITIES (Cold), Iced

ARANEA DIADEMA	
ARSENICUM ALBUM	
CAMPHORA	
CARBO VEGETABILIS	
PHOSPHORUS	
PULSATILLA	*Extremities cold, with body warm*
TABACUM	

SILICEA
VERATRUM ALBUM

FEET (Cold) in bed

CALCAREA CARBONICA — *Sensation of cold and wet stockings*
GRAPHITES — *Sensation of cold and wet stockings*
KALIUM CARBONICUM
PSORINUM
SEPIA
SILICEA

FOOT (One) Hot and the other cold

LYCOPODIUM — *Rarely encountered*
PULSATILLA

HEAD (Cold): Sensation of ice

CALCAREA CARBONICA
VERATRUM ALBUM

SHOULDERS (Cold between the)

ABIES CANADENSIS
AGARICUS MUSCARIUS
LACHNANTES

SWEATING (With Cold)

TABACUM
VERATRUM ALBUM — *Forehead*

WATER Cold

Flowing
AGARICUS MUSCARIUS — *Along the spine*
VERATRUM ALBUM — *In the veins*

Poured on the body
CUPRUM METALLICUM — *Head*
RHUS TOXICODENDRON
VERATRUM ALBUM

COMPRESSION

See **BANDAGE**

CONGESTION

See **POUNDING**

CONSTRICTION

See TIGHTNESS

CONTUSION

See BRUISING

CRACKING NOISES in the ears

HEPAR SULFUR	*When blowing the nose*
KALIUM CARBONICUM	*Auditive hyperesthesia*
KALIUM MURIATICUM	*With eustachian tube catarrh*
NITRICUM ACIDUM	*Auditive hyperesthesia*
PETROLEUM	
SILICEA	

CRAMPS

ACTAEA RACEMOSA (CIMICIFUGA)	*Muscular with involuntary muscle spasms, gynecological*
ALUMINA	*Calves*
ANGUSTURA	*Leg extensors*
ASA FOETIDA	*Esophagus*
AURUM METALLICUM	*Wrists*
CACTUS	*Bladder, uterus, lower limbs*
CHAMOMILLA	
COCCULUS	*Stomach*
COLOCYNTHIS	*Digestive, renal, gynecological*
CUPRUM ARSENICOSUM	*Lower limbs with arterial spasms*
CUPRUM METALLICUM	*Violent, fleeting, digestive and muscular*
CYCLAMEN	
DIOSCOREA	
GELSEMIUM	*Fingers*
GRAPHITES	*Stomach, improved when eating*
LACHESIS MUTUS	*Anus*
MAGNESIA CARBONICA	
MAGNESIA MURIATICA	
MAGNESIA PHOSPHORICA	*Fleeting, digestive, genital, urinary, obstetrical and muscular. Improved by flexing the upper leg towards the pelvis.*
MANGANUM	*Calves*
NATRUM MURIATICUM	*Hyperventilating "terrain"*
NUX VOMICA	*Muscular and visceral with anti-peristaltic effect*
PLATINA	*Localized digestive, gynecological and muscular*
PLUMBUM METALLICUM	
PODOPHYLLUM	*During bowel movement*
SECALE CORNUTUM	*Lower limbs. Improvement when walking on a cold surface*

SULFUR (SULPHUR)	*Calves and soles of the feet*
VERATRUM ALBUM	*Abdominal, of the calves with diarrhea*
VIBURNUM OPULUS	*Of the calves during pregnancy*

CRUSHING PAIN: *"As if the affected areas were pinched between claws" (Neuralgia)*

DIOSCOREA	*Gastric, intestinal, sciatica, uterine*
RANUNCULUS BULBOSUS	*Intercostal neuralgia*
VERBASCUM	*Facial*

DEATH Imminent (Like a premonition)

ACONITUM	*Acute anxiety crisis, with red blood flow, precordial pain*
ARSENICUM ALBUM	*Acute anxiety crisis*
AURUM METALLICUM	*Suicidal*
LATRODECTUS MACTANS	*Coronary attack*
NAJA NAJA (NAJA TRIPUDIANS)	*Coronary attack*
PLATINA	*Hysterical*

DISGUST for food

See **ABSENCE of hunger**

DISLOCATION of the pelvis

See **SPACING OF THE PELVIC BONES**

DIZZINESS

See also **FAINTING SPELLS**

CLOSING the eyes (While)

ALUMINA	
ARGENTUM NITRICUM	
LACHESIS MUTUS	
THERIDION	*Auditive hyperesthesia*

ELDERLY (In the elderly)

ARSENICUM ALBUM
CAUSTICUM
PHOSPHORUS
SULFUR (SULPHUR)

FATIGUE Nervous (Due to)

ARGENTUM NITRICUM	*Anxiety*
COCCULUS	*Lack of sleep*
GELSEMIUM	*Anxiety*
NUX VOMICA	*Too many stimulants*
PHOSPHORICUM ACIDUM	*Moral shock*

Sensations

HEADACHES and visual disorders (With)

CYCLAMEN	*"Transparent" dizziness*
GELSEMIUM	
NATRUM MURIATICUM	
PSORINUM	

HYPOTENSION Orthostatic (Due to)

CHINA (CINCHONA)	
FERRUM METALLICUM	*When sitting down, or going downhill, or if on water*
NATRUM MURIATICUM	
SEPIA	
VERATRUM ALBUM	

LYING DOWN and moving the eyes

CONIUM

MOVEMENT (Due to) of the head and eyes

BRYONIA
COCCULUS
CONIUM
GELSEMIUM

VERTIGO

ARGENTUM NITRICUM	*When looking up at tall buildings*
BORAX	*When looking down*

DRILLING PAIN

AGARICUS MUSCARIUS	
ARGENTUM NITRICUM	
AURUM METALLICUM	*In the bones*
DULCAMARA	*In the joints, muscles and tendons. Sensation of piercing cold*
HEPAR SULFUR	
MERCURIUS SOLUBILIS	*Ocular and in the bones*
SPIGELIA ANTHELMIA	*Migraines and neuralgia*

DROWSINESS

See **SLEEPINESS**

DRYNESS of the mucous membranes

ALUMINA	*Digestive, ocular*
BELLADONNA	
BRYONIA	*All mucous membranes*
CONIUM	*Larynx*

NATRUM MURIATICUM	*Alternating with hypersecretion*
NUX MOSCHATA	*Digestive*
OPIUM	*Diminution of all discharges, except sweat and breast milk*
SANGUINARIA CANADENSIS	*With burning*
SPONGIA	*Larynx*
STICTA PULMONARIA	*Nose and soft palate*
STRAMONIUM	*With fever*

EYES (Of the)

ACONITUM
ALUMINA
ARSENICUM ALBUM
BELLADONNA
BRYONIA
LYCOPODIUM
NUX MOSCHATA
SULFUR (SULPHUR)
ZINCUM METALLICUM

MOUTH (Of the)

Without thirst

APIS
GELSEMIUM — *Classically, absence of thirst; but thirst if there is fever*
NUX MOSCHATA
PULSATILLA

With thirst

ARSENICUM ALBUM
BELLADONNA
BRYONIA
CHAMOMILLA
RHUS TOXICODENDRON
VERATRUM ALBUM

With fever or inflammatory syndrome

APIS
ARNICA
BELLADONNA
BRYONIA
RHUS TOXICODENDRON
STRAMONIUM

ELECTRICAL DISCHARGE

See **POUNDING PAIN**

EMPTINESS

ABDOMEN

COCCULUS

MURIATICUM ACIDUM	
PHOSPHORUS	*And in the head*
PODOPHYLLUM	*After diarrhea*

CHEST (In the)

COCCULUS	
PHOSPHORICUM ACIDUM	
STANNUM METALLICUM	*Aggravation when talking*
SULFUR (SULPHUR)	

STOMACH (In the pit of the): *Need to snack*

KALIUM PHOSPHORICUM

At 10 a.m. (between 9 and 11 a.m.)

KALIUM PHOSPHORICUM
NATRUM MURIATICUM

Around 11 a.m.

IGNATIA
PHOSPHORUS
SEPIA
SULFUR (SULPHUR)
ZINCUM METALLICUM

Not improved when eating

CARBO VEGETABILIS
HYDRASTIS
IGNATIA
SEPIA

ERRATIC PAIN

AESCULUS HIPPOCASTANUM	*Superficial, improved by heat*
BENZOICUM ACIDUM	*In the joints*
BERBERIS	*In the joints*
CAULOPHYLLUM	*Interphalangeal*
COLCHICUM	*In the joints, improved by heat*
FERRUM METALLICUM	*Inflammatory*
FORMICA RUFA	*In the joints*
IGNATIA	*Sudden, fleeting and punctate*
KALIUM BICHROMICUM	*In very limited areas*
KALIUM CARBONICUM	*Throbbing, from area to area, independent of movement*
KALIUM SULFURICUM	*In the joints*
KALMIA	*Neuralgia as by an electric shock; centrifuge*
LAC CANINUM	*Moving from one side to the other*
LYCOPUS	*In the joints*
MAGNESIA PHOSPHORICA	*Spasms and cramps of all types*
PHYTOLACCA	*Sudden, nighttime pain due to damp weather*
PULSATILLA	*Moves quickly*
RADIUM BROMATUM	*In the joints mainly*

RHODODENDRON	*Sensitive to stormy weather*
SULFUR (SULPHUR)	*In the joints*
TUBERCULINUM	*Rheumatic*

EXHALE (Unable to)

DROSERA	*Tracheobronchitis*
SAMBUCUS	*Asthma, laryngitis*

EXHAUSTION

See also **WEAKNESS**

EXHAUSTION after intellectual work

ANACARDIUM ORIENTALE
KALIUM PHOSPHORICUM
NATRUM MURIATICUM
SILICEA

FAINTING SPELL

BATH (In a hot)

LACHESIS MUTUS

GETTING UP (When) From lying down

ACONITUM
BRYONIA
DIGITALIS

HOT FLASH (After a)

SEPIA

HYPERVENTILATION (On "terrain")

MOSCHUS
NUX MOSCHATA

KNEES (When on the)

SEPIA

STANDING UP for a long time (Without sitting down)

FLUORICUM ACIDUM	*Headache*
LILIUM TIGRINUM	
SEPIA	
SULFUR (SULPHUR)	
TUBERCULINUM	

VASO-VAGAL (Due to syndrome)

DIGITALIS
TABACUM
VERATRUM ALBUM

FAINTNESS

See ▸ FAINTING SPELL

FALSE Painful URGE (*Anal and/or bladder tenesmus*)

ARGENTUM NITRICUM	
ARSENICUM ALBUM	
BELLADONNA	
BERBERIS	
CANTHARIS	*Permanent burning urinary tenesmus*
CAPSICUM	*Urinary and rectal tenesmus. Intense burning*
CONIUM	
LACHESIS MUTUS	
LILIUM TIGRINUM	
LYCOPODIUM	
MERCURIUS CORROSIVUS	
MERCURIUS SOLUBILIS	
NITRICUM ACIDUM	
NUX VOMICA	
PAREIRA BRAVA	*Bladder*
PLUMBUM	
PRUNUS SPINOSA	*Bladder*
TEREBINTHINA	*Urinary mostly*
THUYA (THUJA OCCIDENTALIS)	

FALSE URGES

BOWEL MOVEMENTS (With sensation of insufficient stools)

LYCOPODIUM	*Anal spasm, with bloating in the lower abdomen, aggravation when traveling*
NUX VOMICA	*Typical sensation of having incomplete bowel movements, sensation that some matter remains in the rectum after defecating*
PLATINA	*Clay-like stools, aggravation when traveling*
PULSATILLA	
SEPIA	
SILICEA	*With stools that are difficult to expel*
SULFUR (SULPHUR)	
THUYA (THUJA OCCIDENTALIS)	*With stools that are difficult to expel*

URINATE (To): Frequent urges to urinate to no avail

ACONITUM	*In newborn children, due to acute urine retention*
APIS	

CANTHARIS	
CAUSTICUM	
CHIMAPHILA	
CONIUM	*With headache*
HYOSCYAMUS	*With urine retention*
NUX VOMICA	*Painful urinary tenesmus and associated rectal tenesmus*
PLUMBUM	
PULSATILLA	*Mainly when lying on the back*
SARSAPARILLA	*Renal pain on the right*

FATIGUE

See **WEAKNESS**

FEAR felt in the pit of the stomach

CALCAREA CARBONICA
KALIUM CARBONICUM
MEZEREUM
PHOSPHORUS

FILAMENTOUS PAIN

See **LINEAR (Pain)**

FISHBONE

See **THORN**

FLASHING PAIN

See **THROBBING (Pain)**

FOG IN FRONT OF EYES

See **SEE HAZY**

FULLNESS (Painful) of the bladder, not improved by urination

EQUISETUM HIEMALE

GAS (Food turning into)

KALIUM CARBONICUM

GLASS (Sensation of being made of), Fragility

THUYA (THUJA OCCIDENTALIS)

GRAVITY

See **WEIGHT**

Sensations

GRAZE

See WOUND (OPEN WOUND)

HEARING LOSS

CHENOPODIUM ANTHELMINTICUM — *For the human voice, with tinnitus*
CHINA (CINCHONA) — *As if noises were coming from far away*
GRAPHITES — *Hears better if it is noisy nearby*
KALIUM MURIATICUM — *Eustachian tube catarrh. With cracking noises and sensation of obstruction*
KALIUM SULFURICUM
MANGANUM — *Eustachian tube catarrh*
NATRUM MURIATICUM
SILICEA

HEART STOPPING

MOVING (If)

DIGITALIS — *Fear of all movements*

NOT MOVING (If)

GELSEMIUM

SENSATION OF FAINTNESS (With a)

CARBONEUM SULFURATUM

SUFFOCATION (With)

ACTAEA RACEMOSA (CIMICIFUGA)
VIBURNUM OPULUS

VIOLENT SHOCK (Due to): *Extrasystole*

AURUM METALLICUM — *Underlying cardiovascular pathology*
NATRUM MURIATICUM — *Like the fluttering of a bird's wings*

HEAT

See also HOT FLASHES

BODY (Of the entire) With a desire for fresh air

ACONITUM — *Mainly around the head, with boiling sensation, in acute conditions*
BELLADONNA — *Mainly around the head, in acute conditions*
FLUORICUM ACIDUM — *Aggravation due to heat in general*
IODUM — *Intense, permanent*
OPIUM — *Sensation of bed being too hot*
PHOSPHORUS — *Mainly head*

RADIUM BROMATUM	*General burning heat*
SULFUR (SULPHUR)	*Aggravated by the confined heat of the bed*

FACE (Of the) After drinking alcohol

CARBO VEGETABILIS
FLUORICUM ACIDUM

PALMS (Of the) Of the hands

COFFEA TOSTA
PHOSPHORUS
SANGUINARIA CANADENSIS

HEAVINESS

See also **WEIGHT**

EYELIDS (Of the)

BARYTA CARBONICA	
CAUSTICUM	
COCCULUS	
CONIUM	
GELSEMIUM	
LAC CANINUM	
NAJA NAJA (NAJA TRIPUDIANS)	
ONOSMODIUM	
RHUS TOXICODENDRON	
SEPIA	*With left ptosis sometimes*

FOREARMS (Of the)

ARANEA DIADEMA

HEAD (Of the)

CARBO VEGETABILIS	*Like lead, incapable of lifting head from the pillow*
COCCULUS	*Hard to keep head up*
GLONOINUM	*With throbbing*
NAJA NAJA (NAJA TRIPUDIANS)	*With sleepiness and paretic disorders*
NUX MOSCHATA	*With sleepiness*

LEGS (Of the)

Venous origin (Of)

FLUORICUM ACIDUM
HAMAMELIS
PULSATILLA

Weakness (Due to)

GELSEMIUM
PICRICUM ACIDUM

HELMET (*Helmet-like headache*)

IGNATIA

HOT FLASHES

AMYLIUM NITROSUM	*With or without sweating*
ASA FOETIDA	*With palpitations and fainting*
AURUM METALLICUM	
DIGITALIS	
FERRUM METALLICUM	*With usual paleness*
GLONOINUM	*With throbbing of the carotids*
GRAPHITES	*Paleness due to anemia. Sporadic vasomotor hot flashes*
IGNATIA	*Due to emotion*
MELILOTUS OFFICINALIS	*Along with congestive headaches: improved with bleeding*
STRAMONIUM	
SULFUR (SULPHUR)	*With cold feet*
SULFUR IODATUM (SULPHUR IODATUM)	

From chest to head

LACHESIS MUTUS

From hands to head

PHOSPHORUS

From pelvis to head

SEPIA

Of cheeks and ears

SANGUINARIA CANADENSIS

MEAL (After a)

ASA FOETIDA	
CARBO VEGETABILIS	
LYCOPODIUM	*Frequent after lunch*

WINE (Due to drinking)

CARBO VEGETABILIS
LYCOPODIUM
PULSATILLA

HUNGER

ANOREXIA NERVOSA (Alternating with)

CHINA (CINCHONA)

CINA	
FERRUM METALLICUM	
IGNATIA	
LYCOPODIUM	
NATRUM MURIATICUM	*Bulimia, or on the contrary anorexia nervosa*

FEVER (With)

PHOSPHORUS	*During chills*

MIGRAINE (Before or during a)

IGNATIA	*During*
PHOSPHORUS	
PSORINUM	*During*

NIGHT (At)

CHINA (CINCHONA)	
CINA	
FLUORICUM ACIDUM	
LYCOPODIUM	
NATRUM CARBONICUM	*11 p.m.*
PETROLEUM	
PHOSPHORUS	*3 a.m.*
PSORINUM	*3 a.m.*
SULFUR (SULPHUR)	*Sugar*
TUBERCULINUM	*Cold milk*

OBESITY (With)

ALLIUM SATIVUM
AMMONIUM MURIATICUM
ANTIMONIUM CRUDUM
CALCAREA CARBONICA
CAPSICUM
GRAPHITES
STAPHYSAGRIA
SULFUR (SULPHUR)

SATIATED (Quickly)

CHINA (CINCHONA)	
CYCLAMEN	
LYCOPODIUM	*At the first bite*
PSORINUM	
PULSATILLA	*Sensation of food accumulating in the esophagus*
SULFUR (SULPHUR)	

THINNESS (With)

ABROTANUM
FLUORICUM ACIDUM
IODUM
KALIUM PHOSPHORICUM

Sensations

NATRUM MURIATICUM
PHOSPHORUS
SULFUR IODATUM (SULPHUR IODATUM)
TUBERCULINUM

HYPERIDEATION when going to bed, with insomnia

ACTAEA RACEMOSA (CIMICIFUGA)	
	Plethora of images, as a kaleidoscope
CALCAREA CARBONICA	*Hypersensitivity*
COFFEA TOSTA	*Pursuant to happy emotions, sensorial hypersensitivity, with excitement during the day and mood swings*
GELSEMIUM	*Pursuant to bad news, anticipation anxiety*
NUX VOMICA	*Due to too many stimulants*
STRAMONIUM	*After laughing too much*

HYPERSENSITIVITY

In general

AMBRA GRISEA	*General feeling of discomfort and insomnia*
COFFEA TOSTA	*Sensorial, and to pain*

CONTACT (At the slightest)

See also TOUCH

APIS	
BELLADONNA	
BRYONIA	*Sensitive to the slightest touch*
CHINA (CINCHONA)	*Mostly on the scalp*
CINA	
COFFEA TOSTA	
HEPAR SULFUR	*Mostly on the inflamed areas*
LACHESIS MUTUS	*Very pronounced, associated with intolerance to any constriction*
MAGNESIA CARBONICA	
MERCURIUS SOLUBILIS	
NUX VOMICA	*Mostly when digesting*

CONTRARIETY (At the slightest)

ANTIMONIUM CRUDUM	*Sulks*
AURUM METALLICUM	*Violent anger*
CHAMOMILLA	*Tantrums, sobbing spasms*
CINA	
LYCOPODIUM	*Rare but violent tantrums, vindictive*
NITRICUM ACIDUM	
NUX VOMICA	*Easily angered, impatient, often aggressive*
STAPHYSAGRIA	*Pent-up anger*

DRAFTS (To) Of cold air

CALCAREA CARBONICA	
CHINA (CINCHONA)	*Neuralgia*
HEPAR SULFUR	*Acute Suppuration*
KALIUM CARBONICUM	
NUX VOMICA	*Coryza*
PSORINUM	*Respiratory weakness*
RUMEX	*Cough due to inhaling cold air*
SILICEA	*Respiratory weakness*
TUBERCULINUM	*Respiratory weakness*

EMOTIONS (To happy)

COFFEA TOSTA	*With insomnia when trying to fall asleep*

LIGHT (To): *Photophobia*

ACONITUM	*Acute conjunctivitis after dry cold, exposure to sun reflecting on snow*
ARGENTUM NITRICUM	*After eye strain; purulent conjunctivitis*
ARSENICUM ALBUM	
BELLADONNA	
CALCAREA CARBONICA	
CHINA (CINCHONA)	*Daylight and sunlight*
CONIUM	
EUPHRASIA	*Allergic conjunctivitis*
GRAPHITES	*Daylight and sunlight*
LACHESIS MUTUS	
MERCURIUS CORROSIVUS	
MERCURIUS SOLUBILIS	
NATRUM MURIATICUM	
NATRUM SULFURICUM	*With headache when looking at light*
NUX VOMICA	
OPIUM	
PHOSPHORUS	
PSORINUM	*Hay fever*
RHUS TOXICODENDRON	
SULFUR (SULPHUR)	
TARENTULA HISPANA	*General sensorial hypersensitivity*
ZINCUM METALLICUM	

MUSIC (To)

AMBRA GRISEA	*Head congestion, coughing*
NATRUM SULFURICUM	
PHOSPHORICUM ACIDUM	
PHOSPHORUS	
SABINA	*Nervous agitation*
TARENTULA HISPANA	*With sweating. Contested pathogenesis*

With crying

AMBRA GRISEA
GRAPHITES
NATRUM CARBONICUM
THUYA (THUJA OCCIDENTALIS)

NOISE (To)

ACONITUM	
ACTAEA RACEMOSA (CIMICIFUGA)	
AURUM METALLICUM	
BELLADONNA	*Mainly when feverish*
BORAX	
CAPSICUM	
CAUSTICUM	
CHINA (CINCHONA)	*Evolving towards hypoacusis. Often associated tinnitus*
COCCULUS	
CONIUM	
FERRUM METALLICUM	*Asthenia*
GLONOINUM	
IGNATIA	*But sleeps better when there is noise*
IODUM	
The KALIUM group	*Mostly KALIUM CARBONICUM*
LAC CANINUM	
LACHESIS MUTUS	
LYCOPODIUM	
MAGNESIA CARBONICA	
The NATRUM group	*NATRUM CARBONICUM Particularly sensitive to sudden noises*
NITRICUM ACIDUM	*Sensitive at the same time to shaking and vibrations*
NUX VOMICA	*To familiar noises around the house making patient aggressive*
PHOSPHORICUM ACIDUM	*With aggravation of the headache*
SANGUINARIA CANADENSIS	*During headache*
SILICEA	
SULFUR (SULPHUR)	
ZINCUM METALLICUM	*Mostly hypersensitive to conversations. The slightest noise is startling*

At the slightest noise (crinkling)

ASARUM EUROPAEUM	*High or scratching, sheet of paper, silky material*
COFFEA TOSTA	*Hears noises that others do not*
OPIUM	*Hyperesthesia of all senses but mostly auditive. Hears noises before anyone else.*
THERIDION	*Intolerance to slight noises which seem to penetrate the entire body.*

ODORS (To)

In general

AURUM METALLICUM

BELLADONNA	
CHAMOMILLA	
CHINA (CINCHONA)	
COFFEA TOSTA	*Pronounced hyperosmia*
COLCHICUM	*Disgust and nausea for fish and eggs*
GRAPHITES	
IGNATIA	
LYCOPODIUM	
NUX MOSCHATA	
NUX VOMICA	
PHOSPHORUS	*During a headache*
SEPIA	*Cannot stand the sight of food or smell of cooking, mainly during pregnancy*
SULFUR (SULPHUR)	
Of flowers	
GRAPHITES	
IGNATIA	
NUX VOMICA	
LAC CANINUM	
PHOSPHORUS	
SABADILLA	*And of garlic*
SANGUINARIA CANADENSIS	
Of food	
ARSENICUM ALBUM	
COCCULUS	
COLCHICUM	
IPECA (IPECAC)	
SEPIA	

PAIN (To)

ACONITUM	*With anxious agitation, with a sensation of imminent death*
AURUM METALLICUM	*With suicidal tendencies*
CHAMOMILLA	*With agitation and crying*
COFFEA TOSTA	
HEPAR SULFUR	*Suppurative process*
HYPERICUM	*Neuralgic pain*
IGNATIA	*With paradoxical modalities, improved by distraction*
LACHESIS MUTUS	*Local infection*
NITRICUM ACIDUM	*With splinter-like pain*
NUX MOSCHATA	*With fainting spells*
NUX VOMICA	*With irritability*
PHOSPHORUS	
SILICEA	
STAPHYSAGRIA	*Pursuant to cuts or wounds*
THUYA (THUJA OCCIDENTALIS)	*With suicidal tendencies*

TICKLING (To)

KALIUM CARBONICUM
PHOSPHORUS

TOUCH (To)

See also **HYPERSENSITIVITY to contact**

Of the breast

LAC CANINUM
SILICEA

Of the chest

CURARE

Of the costal-lumbar angle

BERBERIS	*Left*
SOLIDAGO	*Right*

Of the feet

KALIUM CARBONICUM	*Jumps when startled*

Of the genital organs

ACTAEA RACEMOSA (CIMICIFUGA)	
MURIATICUM ACIDUM	*And hemorrhoids*

- With sexual arousal

MOSCHUS
MUREX
ORIGANUM
PLATINA
STAPHYSAGRIA

In inflammatory and infectious states

APIS	
ARNICA	
ASA FOETIDA	*Except abdominal pain*
BELLADONNA	
BRYONIA	
CANTHARIS	
HEPAR SULFUR	
LACHESIS MUTUS	
TEREBINTHINA	*Of the abdomen with bloating*
VERATRUM ALBUM	*Abdomen*

Of the limbs

MANGANUM	
TARENTULA HISPANA	*Fingertips*
THALLIUM ACETICUM	

Of the mucous membranes of the mouth

COCCUS CACTI	*Nausea*

Of the neck (with intolerance to constriction around the neck)

ARGENTUM NITRICUM	
CALCAREA CARBONICA	
CENCHRIS	
LACHESIS MUTUS	*With sensation of choking, intolerance to any tight clothes, hot flashes*

NAJA NAJA (NAJA TRIPUDIANS)	
SEPIA	*With hot flashes*

Of the scalp, hair (when brushing)

AMBRA GRISEA	*Sensation of wound*
BELLADONNA	
CARBO VEGETABILIS	*Intolerance to wearing a hat*
CAUSTICUM	*Sensation of hair being pulled out*
CHINA (CINCHONA)	
COFFEA TOSTA	
FERRUM METALLICUM	
HEPAR SULFUR	
NITRICUM ACIDUM	
NUX VOMICA	*Occiput*
PHOSPHORUS	*Sensation of hair being pulled out*
SILICEA	*While brushing ones hair*
SULFUR (SULPHUR)	

Of the spine

ACTAEA RACEMOSA (CIMICIFUGA)	*T3 to T8 (= 3rd to 8th thoracic vertebra)*
LAC CANINUM	
PHOSPHORUS	*On impact to the thoracic vertebras*
SILICEA	*Coccyx*
TELLURIUM	*Spine*
ZINCUM METALLICUM	*Neck and dorsolumbar joint*

Of the sub-sternal notch (with coughing)

HYDRASTIS
RUMEX

Of the waist (tight belt)

CHINA (CINCHONA)
CROTALUS HORRIDUS
GRAPHITES
LACHESIS MUTUS
LYCOPODIUM
NATRUM SULFURICUM
NUX VOMICA

HYPOACUSIS

See **HEARING LOSS**

ICE

See **COLD**

IDEAS (FLOW OF IDEAS)

See **HYPERIDEATION**

INDIFFERENCE Affective

ANACARDIUM ORIENTALE	*Due to nervous fatigue, with memory loss, indecisive*

FLUORICUM ACIDUM	*Due to affective instability*
KALIUM BROMATUM	*Due to intellectual overexertion*
LYCOPODIUM	*To ones own children; keeps them at a distance*
PHOSPHORICUM ACIDUM	*Indifferent to everything, due to nervous exhaustion*
PHOSPHORUS	
PICRICUM ACIDUM	*Due to nervous exhaustion*
PLATINA	*Depression*
SEPIA	*To everything and everyone*

INHALE Deeply (Need to)

See LACK OF AIR

INSECTS crawling on skin

See TINGLING

INSOMNIA

See HYPERIDEATION

INSTABILITY When walking

See DIZZINESS

INTOLERANCE (To)

See HYPERSENSITIVITY

IRON CLAMP

See TIGHTNESS

ITCHING

See PRURITUS

KNEES Giving out

See WEAKNESS

LACK OF AIR, Need to inhale deeply, to sigh

See also CHOKING

IGNATIA	*With lump in throat*
LACHESIS MUTUS	*Intolerance to constriction of the neck*
MOSCHUS	*With fainting*

LACK OF STRENGTH

See WEAKNESS

LIBIDO increase

See AROUSAL sexual

LIGHTNESS of the limbs

ASARUM EUROPAEUM	*Rarely encountered. Auditive hypersensitivity is more frequent*

LINEAR PAINS

ALLIUM CEPA	*Filiform pain along the nerves, eustachian tube*
CAPSICUM	
LUESINUM (SYPHILINUM)	*In the bones*
OXALICUM ACIDUM	*Aggravation when thinking about it*

LIPOTHYMIA

See FAINTING SPELL

LISP (Speech impediment)

KALIUM BICHROMICUM	*Base of the tongue*
NATRUM MURIATICUM	*With a sensation of dryness*
NATRUM PHOSPHORICUM	*Tip of the tongue*
SILICEA	*Anterior part*

LOSS of smell

See ABSENCE of olfaction

LOSS of taste

See ABSENCE of taste

LUMP

BLADDER (Near the)

ANACARDIUM ORIENTALE	
LACHESIS MUTUS	*Lump rolling around the lower abdomen and bladder*

CARDIA (Near the)

ABIES NIGRA	*Esophageal spasm, with sensation of an egg stuck there*

Sensations

ESOPHAGUS (Near the)

ASA FOETIDA	*Mobile, bottom to top*
IGNATIA	
LACHESIS MUTUS	
MOSCHUS	*Identical to IGNATIA on a pronounced hysterical "terrain"*
SEPIA	
VALERIANA	

PERINEAL REGION (Near the)

CHIMAPHILA	*Sitting, for a prostatic patient*

RECTUM (In the)

ANACARDIUM ORIENTALE	*"Plugged" sensation*
LACHESIS MUTUS	
SEPIA	*Persistent after bowel movement*

STOMACH (Near the), rising in the throat

ASA FOETIDA
PLUMBUM
SUMBUL
ZINCUM METALLICUM

THROAT (Near the)

IGNATIA	*With need to inhale deeply*
LACHESIS MUTUS	*With choking*
SEPIA	
SUMBUL	

MOOD Changing

See **VARIABLE mood**

NAIL planted in the head

AGARICUS MUSCARIUS	*Right temple*
COFFEA TOSTA	*Parietal*
HEPAR SULFUR	
IGNATIA	*Parietal and occipital*
NUX VOMICA	*Vertex*
SEPIA	
THUYA (THUJA OCCIDENTALIS)	*Frontal*

NAUSEA

In general

ANTIMONIUM CRUDUM	*White tongue*
ANTIMONIUM TARTARICUM	*Symptomatic triad: paleness, fatigue, sleepiness*

ARGENTUM NITRICUM	*With eructation, aggravation due to sweets*
ARSENICUM ALBUM	*Acute gastroenteritis*
BRYONIA	*At the slightest movement*
COCCULUS	*Motion sickness*
COCCUS CACTI	*When brushing teeth*
COLCHICUM	*At the slightest sight, odor or thought of food*
CUPRUM METALLICUM	*With cramping pain*
DIGITALIS	*Clean tongue*
IPECA (IPECAC)	*Clean tongue*
IRIS VERSICOLOR	*With pyrosis*
KALIUM CARBONICUM	*With generalized bloating*
LOBELIA	*With vaso-vagal syndrome*
NUX VOMICA	*Improved by vomiting; forced vomiting sometimes*
PETROLEUM	*Improved by eating*
PULSATILLA	*With intolerance to fatty foods*
SEPIA	*Improved after breakfast*
SULFUR (SULPHUR)	*Brought on by ones own body odor*
TABACUM	*With vaso-vagal syndrome*
VERATRUM ALBUM	*With vaso-vagal syndrome, cold sweating*

CLEAN TONGUE (With)

ASARUM EUROPAEUM
DIGITALIS
IPECA (IPECAC)

HYPERSALIVATION (With))

COCCULUS
LACTICUM ACIDUM
LOBELIA
MERCURIUS SOLUBILIS
NUX VOMICA
PETROLEUM
TABACUM

INTENSE, SYNCOPAL

COCCULUS
DIGITALIS
IPECA (IPECAC)
KALIUM CARBONICUM
LACHESIS MUTUS
LOBELIA
NUX VOMICA
PULSATILLA
TABACUM

MOTION SICKNESS (With)

COCCULUS
NUX MOSCHATA
NUX VOMICA

PETROLEUM
SEPIA
STAPHYSAGRIA
TABACUM

ODORS (Due to)

COCCULUS
COLCHICUM
DIGITALIS
EUPATORIUM PERFOLIATUM
PHOSPHORICUM ACIDUM
SEPIA
STANNUM METALLICUM

PREGNANCY (Of)

ACTAEA RACEMOSA (CIMICIFUGA)	
ANACARDIUM ORIENTALE	*Improved by eating*
ARSENICUM ALBUM	
IGNATIA	
KALIUM CARBONICUM	*With burping and heartburn*
KREOSOTUM	
LACTICUM ACIDUM	
LOBELIA	
MERCURIUS SOLUBILIS	
NUX VOMICA	
SEPIA	*Before breakfast, when rinsing the mouth*
SYMPHORICARPUS	
TABACUM	*With hypersalivation, improved when breathing fresh air*

NEED to DEFECATE or URINATE

See **URGE**

NEEDLES (Pain like needles)

See **THROBBING (Pain)**

NEURALGIA (Pain)

See **THROBBING (Pain)**

NUMBNESS

In general

ASA FOETIDA	
CARBONEUM SULFURATUM	*Localized hypoesthesia or paresthesia*
COCCULUS	

Alternating with pain

GNAPHALIUM POLYCEPHALUM	*Cruralgia, femoral paresthesia*

Of the extremities: *Acroparesthesia*

ARANEA DIADEMA	*Fourth and fifth digits of the hand (nerve path C8-T1)*
COCCULUS	*Mainly upper limbs*
DIGITALIS	
FLUORICUM ACIDUM	
LATRODECTUS MACTANS	*Associated with intense mid-chest pain*
OXALICUM ACIDUM	*Often associated with characteristic linear pain*
PHOSPHORUS	

Of the lower limbs when resting

ALUMINA	
AMBRA GRISEA	*Arms*
ARANEA DIADEMA	*Forearms*
GRAPHITES	
PULSATILLA	

With pain

ABROTANUM	*Chilblains*
ACONITUM	*Left arm, with hand paresis*
ASA FOETIDA	*Hyperventilation "terrain"*
CHAMOMILLA	*Or after pain*
CONIUM	
KALIUM CARBONICUM	*When lying down*
KALMIA	*Associated with sudden centrifugal neuralgia*
MAGNESIA PHOSPHORICA	*Parts of the body one is resting on*
PLATINA	
RHUS TOXICODENDRON	*Like MAGNESIA PHOSPHORICA*
VERBASCUM	

OBSTRUCTION

EARS (Of the)

KALIUM MURIATICUM
MERCURIUS DULCIS
SILICEA

LARYNX (Of the)

SPONGIA

NOSE (Of the)

AMMONIUM CARBONICUM	*In the newborn, with crusting*
AURUM METALLICUM	*With sinusitis*
DULCAMARA	*Due to humidity*
LYCOPODIUM	*Chronic*
MANGANUM	

NUX VOMICA	*At night, due to heat*
SAMBUCUS	
STICTA PULMONARIA	*With dryness and sensation of pressure at the base of the nose*

In spite of nasal discharge

AMMONIUM MURIATICUM	
ARSENICUM ALBUM	
KALIUM SULFURICUM	*Green*
PULSATILLA	*Green*
SABADILLA	

OPPRESSION thoracic or respiratory

See **CHOKING**

PALPITATIONS

See **POUNDING heart**

PERIODS Imminent

ONOSMODIUM	
PLATINA	
SENECIO AUREUS	*Late or suppressed menstruation with vicariate bleeding*

PHOTOPHOBIA

See **HYPERSENSITIVITY to light**

PLUG

ANACARDIUM ORIENTALE	*In the anus*
ASARUM EUROPAEUM	*In the ears*
NAJA NAJA (NAJA TRIPUDIANS)	*In the esophagus*
SABADILLA	*In the throat*

POINT (Pain localized at one particular point)

See **PUNCTATE (Pain)**

POLLAKIURIA

See **frequent URGE to URINATE**

POUNDING, pulsation, local congestion (Blood flow)

AMBRA GRISEA	*Moves up the limbs*
AURUM METALLICUM	
BELLADONNA	*Concomitant to local and general congestion*
CHINA (CINCHONA)	

DIGITALIS	
FERRUM METALLICUM	*Pounding in the entire body, like little hammers*
GLONOINUM	
IODUM	*In the entire body*
KALIUM CARBONICUM	*Due to anemia*
LACHESIS MUTUS	*Improved by any discharge*
NATRUM MURIATICUM	*In the entire body*
PHOSPHORUS	
STRONTIUM CARBONICUM	*Improved by heat*
SULFUR (SULPHUR)	

ANUS (Of the)

AESCULUS HIPPOCASTANUM	
LACHESIS MUTUS	*Like little hammers, with a constricted sensation*

HEAD (Of the)

ASTERIAS RUBENS	*Permanent or intermittent congestion with face red*
BELLADONNA	
CACTUS	*With heat*
CALCAREA CARBONICA	*With sensation of external cold*
CHINA (CINCHONA)	*From one temple to the other or occipital*
FERRUM METALLICUM	*Pale face with vasomotor flashes*
GELSEMIUM	*Headaches and migraines during flu syndromes and sunburn/sunstroke*
GLONOINUM	*Synchroneity of the pulse with a bursting sensation*
GRAPHITES	*Pale face, cold body with vasomotor flashes*
LACHESIS MUTUS	
MELILOTUS OFFICINALIS	*Sensation that blood is going to burst out from all orifices, improved by blood flow*
NATRUM MURIATICUM	*Like little hammers pounding the brain*
OPIUM	*Face red and congested without pain*
PHYTOLACCA	*With a sensation of cold in the rest of the body*
PULSATILLA	
SANGUINARIA CANADENSIS	*Congestive headache. Menstrual migraines. Hot flashes*
SEPIA	*Suborbital migraine on the left side*
STRAMONIUM	*Violent congestive headaches. With only one painful area*
VERATRUM VIRIDE	*Intense cephalic congestion with relative bradycardia*

HEART (Of the)

ACONITUM	*Tachycardia with hard and tense pulse. Bouts of arterial hypertension*
AMBRA GRISEA	*Of emotional origin*
ARGENTUM NITRICUM	*Lying on the right side*
CACTUS	*With a sensation of constriction*
COFFEA TOSTA	
IGNATIA	*Emotional*
IODUM	*Palpitations at the slightest effort*

LACHESIS MUTUS
LILIUM TIGRINUM — *Functional arrhythmia on a neurotic "terrain"*
LYCOPUS — *Very fast and violent beating of the heart*
NAJA NAJA (NAJA TRIPUDIANS) — *Bradyarrythmia aggravated when lying on the left side and when talking*
NATRUM MURIATICUM
SPIGELIA ANTHELMIA — *Violent palpitations perceptible through clothes*

INFLAMED AREAS (Of the)

BELLADONNA
LACHESIS MUTUS

NECK (Of the)

ACONITUM
ARGENTUM NITRICUM
AURUM METALLICUM
CACTUS
GLONOINUM
LACHESIS MUTUS

PRESSURE

HEAD, EYES, LIMBS, CHEST (On the)

PHOSPHORICUM ACIDUM

NOSE (At the root of the)

During epistaxis

CHINA (CINCHONA)
HAMAMELIS

During ENT infections

CINNABARIS (MERCURIUS SULPHURATUS RUBER) — *At the base of the nose, just like glasses*
GELSEMIUM
IODUM — *With coryza or headache*
KALIUM BICHROMICUM
KALIUM IODATUM
STICTA PULMONARIA

PRICKLING

See **TINGLING**

PRURITUS

In general

AGARICUS MUSCARIUS	*Chilblains*
ANACARDIUM ORIENTALE	*Improved by eating*
APIS	*Skin rash*
ARSENICUM ALBUM	
CALCAREA CARBONICA	*Cephalic eczema with pruritus when waking up*
CAUSTICUM	
DOLICHOS PRURIENS	
FAGOPYRUM	*Hairy areas, eyes, anus, palms of the hands; senescent, allergic, aggravated between 4 and 8 p.m. and by heat, like LYCOPODIUM*
FLUORICUM ACIDUM	
GRAPHITES	
KALIUM SULFURICUM	*Squamous on a wet base, or suppurating eruptions*
LEDUM PALUSTRE	
LYCOPODIUM	
MANGANUM	*Of the skin folds, aggravated by sweating*
MERCURIUS SOLUBILIS	
MEZEREUM	
NATRUM MURIATICUM	
PETROLEUM	
PSORINUM	
PULSATILLA	
RHUS TOXICODENDRON	
SEPIA	
SILICEA	
STAPHYSAGRIA	
SULFUR (SULPHUR)	
URTICA URENS	*Skin rash, aggravation by water*

ANUS (Of the)

AESCULUS HIPPOCASTANUM	
ALOE	
CALCAREA CARBONICA	
CAUSTICUM	
CINA	*Aggravation at night, and when the moon is full*
COLLINSONIA	
FLUORICUM ACIDUM	
GRAPHITES	
KALIUM CARBONICUM	
LYCOPODIUM	
NATRUM MURIATICUM	
NITRICUM ACIDUM	
NUX VOMICA	
PAEONIA	
PETROLEUM	
PULSATILLA	

RATANHIA
SEPIA
SILICEA
STAPHYSAGRIA
SULFUR (SULPHUR)
TEUCRIUM MARUM
THUYA (THUJA OCCIDENTALIS)
ZINCUM METALLICUM

ANUS (Of the) and of the NOSE

CINA	*Oxyurosis*
TEUCRIUM MARUM	*Oxyurosis, nasal polyposis*

EARS (Of the)

With otorrhea

AURUM METALLICUM
HEPAR SULFUR
TELLURIUM

With chilblains (redness and burning)

AGARICUS MUSCARIUS
PETROLEUM

ERRATIC

MANGANUM
MEZEREUM
STAPHYSAGRIA

EUSTACHIAN TUBE (Of the)

ARUNDO DONAX	
CALCAREA CARBONICA	
GELSEMIUM	*With coughing*
NUX VOMICA	*With need to swallow*
PETROLEUM	
SILICEA	

EYELIDS (Of the)

ALUMINA	*Dry eye syndrome*
ARGENTUM METALLICUM	*Blepharo-conjunctivitis*
CALCAREA CARBONICA	
GRAPHITES	
NATRUM SULFURICUM	
PULSATILLA	
RHUS TOXICODENDRON	
SEPIA	
STAPHYSAGRIA	
SULFUR (SULPHUR)	

HAIRY (Of the hairy areas)

FAGOPYRUM	*And of the hands*

HANDS (Of the)

AGARICUS MUSCARIUS	*Chilblains*
ANACARDIUM ORIENTALE	*Improved by eating*
ANAGALLIS	*Palmar and digital dyshidrosis*
FAGOPYRUM	*Palms of the hands*
KALIUM PHOSPHORICUM	*Palms of the hands and soles of the feet*
PETROLEUM	*Aggravated in winter*
PIX LIQUIDA	*Eczema with cracking, and heavy pruritus*
RANUNCULUS BULBOSUS	*Palms of the hands*
SULFUR (SULPHUR)	

NIGHT (At), with the heat of the bed

CARBO VEGETABILIS	*Varicose ulcers*
CLEMATIS ERECTA	*Occiput and edge of the scalp, aggravated by cold water*
DOLICHOS PRURIENS	*Without eruption, senescent, allergic, post-herpetic*
GRAPHITES	
KALIUM ARSENICOSUM	*Squamous eruptions, elbows and knees, aggravated by undressing and by the heat of the bed*
KALIUM PHOSPHORICUM	*Palms of the hands and soles of the feet, improved by soft rubbing*
LEDUM PALUSTRE	*Feet and ankles, rosacea*
LYCOPODIUM	
MERCURIUS SOLUBILIS	*When sweating*
MEZEREUM	*Vesicular eruptions first purulent then scabby, whitish pus*
PSORINUM	*In the winter*
PULSATILLA	*Generalized pruritus; skin rash after fatty foods*
SULFUR (SULPHUR)	

NIPPLES (Of the)

FLUORICUM ACIDUM
GRAPHITES
ORIGANUM
PETROLEUM
SULFUR (SULPHUR)

NOSE (Of the)

ARUM TRIPHYLLUM	
ARUNDO DONAX	*As well as the soft palate and the auditory tubes*
CINA	*Feels need to constantly put fingers up nose*
NUX VOMICA	*Inside of the nose*
RANUNCULUS BULBOSUS	

SABADILLA
SILICEA
SUCCINICUM ACIDUM — *And of the eyelids; asthma*
SULFUR (SULPHUR)
TEUCRIUM MARUM

ORIFICES Cutaneous mucous (Of the)

FLUORICUM ACIDUM
NITRICUM ACIDUM
SULFUR (SULPHUR)

SCALP (Of the)

AGARICUS MUSCARIUS
ARSENICUM ALBUM
BARYTA CARBONICA — *Nape of neck*
CICUTA VIROSA
GRAPHITES
LYCOPODIUM
MEZEREUM
OLEANDER
SULFUR (SULPHUR)
VIOLA TRICOLOR

SCARS (Of the)

CALCAREA FLUORICA
FLUORICUM ACIDUM

SENILE

ALUMINA
AMBRA GRISEA
ARSENICUM ALBUM
DOLICHOS PRURIENS
FAGOPYRUM
PSORINUM
RADIUM BROMATUM
SULFUR (SULPHUR)

"SINE MATERIA" (= Without eruption)

ALUMINA
AMBRA GRISEA
ARSENICUM ALBUM
DOLICHOS PRURIENS — *With jaundice or constipation*
FAGOPYRUM
MEDORRHINUM
MERCURIUS SOLUBILIS
MEZEREUM
PETROLEUM
PSORINUM

PULSATILLA
RADIUM BROMATUM
STAPHYSAGRIA — *Changes places when scratched*
SULFUR (SULPHUR)

SOFT PALATE (Of the)

SABADILLA — *And of the nose*
WYETHIA

SOFT PALATE (Of the), Of the ears (Eustachian tube) and of the nose

ARUNDO DONAX

SUN (After exposure to the): *Benign summer light eruption (BSLE)*

FAGOPYRUM
HYPERICUM
MURIATICUM ACIDUM
NATRUM MURIATICUM
PULSATILLA

UNDRESSING (When)

ARSENICUM ALBUM
KALIUM ARSENICOSUM
KALIUM BICHROMICUM
MEDORRHINUM
NATRUM SULFURICUM
OLEANDER
RADIUM BROMATUM
RUMEX — *And with cold air*
TUBERCULINUM

URINARY MEATUS (Of the)

PETROSELINUM SATIVUM — *Navicular fossa*
SULFUR (SULPHUR) — *With redness*

VARICOSE VEINS (Of the) and varicose ulcers

FLUORICUM ACIDUM

VULVO VAGINAL

AMBRA GRISEA — *Psychosomatic*
COFFEA TOSTA — *With hyperesthesia to the touch*
CONIUM — *During and after menstruation*
CROTON TIGLIUM — *Intense pruritus improved by soft rubbing*
FLUORICUM ACIDUM — *Pruritus at the orifices, aggravated by heat, like SULFUR (SULPHUR)*
GRAPHITES — *Pruritus of the vulva before menstruation*

MERCURIUS SOLUBILIS	*During menstruation*
PETROLEUM	
RHUS TOXICODENDRON	
SARSAPARILLA	
SEPIA	
SULFUR (SULPHUR)	

With sexual arousal ("voluptuous" pruritus)

AMBRA GRISEA	
CALADIUM	*In pregnant women*
COFFEA TOSTA	
KREOSOTUM	
LILIUM TIGRINUM	
ORIGANUM	*With pruritus of the nipples*
PLATINA	*With hyperesthesia to the touch*
SULFUR (SULPHUR)	
ZINCUM METALLICUM	

With leukorrhea

CALCAREA CARBONICA	
GRAPHITES	
HELONIAS DIOICA	
KREOSOTUM	
MERCURIUS SOLUBILIS	
NATRUM MURIATICUM	*Alternating with vaginal dryness*
NITRICUM ACIDUM	
PETROLEUM	
PULSATILLA	
SEPIA	
SILICEA	
SULFUR (SULPHUR)	

WARTS (Of the)

SABINA	*Localized in the genital/anal area, bleeding*
SEPIA	

PULSATING PAIN

See THROBBING PAIN

PULSATION

See POUNDING

PUNCTATE PAIN

ACTAEA RACEMOSA (CIMICIFUGA)	*Under the left breast*
BRYONIA	*At the slightest movement*
COFFEA TOSTA	*Spike-like sensation*

IGNATIA	*And erratic*
KALIUM BICHROMICUM	
KALIUM CARBONICUM	*Independent of movement*
KALIUM SULFURICUM	*And erratic*
MOSCHUS	*Under the left breast*
THUYA (THUJA OCCIDENTALIS)	*Spike-like sensation*

RESTLESSNESS of the lower limbs "fidgety legs"

ARSENICUM ALBUM	
CAUSTICUM	*With rheumatoid disorders*
KALIUM CARBONICUM	
LYCOPODIUM	
MEDORRHINUM	*Painful*
NATRUM MURIATICUM	
PLATINA	
SULFUR (SULPHUR)	
ZINCUM METALLICUM	*Very asthenic but highly pronounced osteo-tendinous reflexes*

SATIATED (Quickly)

See **HUNGER QUICKLY SATIATED**

SEARING PAIN

See **THROBBING (PAIN)**

SEE (To)

See also **WEAKNESS of sight**

ANIMALS Figment of imagination

OPIUM

BIGGER (Objects seem larger than usual)

CAUSTICUM
HYOSCYAMUS

COLORS

CHINA (CINCHONA)
CONIUM
PHOSPHORUS

DOUBLE

AGARICUS MUSCARIUS

AURUM METALLICUM	
CHINA (CINCHONA)	
CYCLAMEN	
GELSEMIUM	*During headaches*
HYOSCYAMUS	
NAJA NAJA (NAJA TRIPUDIANS)	
NATRUM MURIATICUM	
NITRICUM ACIDUM	

FRIGHTENING IMAGES

BELLADONNA
CALCAREA CARBONICA
HYOSCYAMUS
KALIUM BROMATUM
LACHESIS MUTUS
SECALE CORNUTUM
STRAMONIUM

FUZZY (Sight) Before a headache (Ophthalmic migraine)

CAUSTICUM	
CYCLAMEN	*Catamenial migraine, with dizziness and visual disorders*
GELSEMIUM	
IRIS VERSICOLOR	
KALIUM BICHROMICUM	*Suborbital migraine on the right side with punctate pain*
LAC DEFLORATUM	*Constipation, intolerance to milk*
LYCOPODIUM	*Right vertical hemianopsia: the patient can only see the left half of the objects*
NATRUM MURIATICUM	*Depending on the solar cycle*
PODOPHYLLUM	
PSORINUM	
SEPIA	
SILICEA	
SULFUR (SULPHUR)	

GHOSTS and spirits during delirium due to hyperthermia

BELLADONNA
LACHESIS MUTUS

HALF (Only the left half of the objects)

LITHIUM CARBONICUM
LYCOPODIUM

HALF (Only the lower half of the objects)

ARSENICUM ALBUM
AURUM METALLICUM
DIGITALIS

HALO Colored, around lights

BELLADONNA
PHOSPHORUS

HAZY

ARSENICUM ALBUM	
BARYTA CARBONICA	
CALCAREA CARBONICA	
CARBONEUM SULFURATUM	*Optic nerve neuritis*
CAUSTICUM	*Cataracts*
CHINA (CINCHONA)	
CONIUM	
CYCLAMEN	
GELSEMIUM	*Often before migraines*
MERCURIUS SOLUBILIS	
NAPHTALINUM	*Cataracts*
NATRUM MURIATICUM	*During or before migraines. Cataracts*
PHOSPHORUS	
PHYSOSTIGMA	
PULSATILLA	
RHUS TOXICODENDRON	
SULFUR (SULPHUR)	
ZINCUM METALLICUM	

HOUSES or walls crushing him

ARGENTUM NITRICUM *During dizziness*

SMALLER (Objects seem smaller than usual)

NUX MOSCHATA
PLATINA

SPARKLES

BELLADONNA
CHINA (CINCHONA)
CYCLAMEN
PHOSPHORUS

SPARKS or flames

BELLADONNA
PHOSPHORUS

STAINS or black dots

CHINA (CINCHONA)
COCCULUS
KALIUM CARBONICUM
LYCOPODIUM
NATRUM MURIATICUM

Sensations

PHOSPHORUS
PHYSOSTIGMA

VISUAL FIELD (Becoming smaller)

GELSEMIUM
NATRUM MURIATICUM

ZIGZAGS

NATRUM MURIATICUM

SHAKING Muscular (Jolts, fasciculation, myoclonus)

ACTAEA RACEMOSA (CIMICIFUGA)	
AGARICUS MUSCARIUS	*Tics*
ANACARDIUM ORIENTALE	*With cramping*
ARGENTUM NITRICUM	*With shaking, paralysis*
ARSENICUM ALBUM	*When going to sleep*
BELLADONNA	*Convulsions*
CHAMOMILLA	
CICUTA VIROSA	*Convulsions*
CINA	*Convulsions*
CUPRUM METALLICUM	*Cramping, convulsions with thumbs flexed inside the palms of the hands*
FLUORICUM ACIDUM	*With agitation of the extremities*
HYOSCYAMUS	*Hands and feet*
IGNATIA	*Eyelids, lips*
KALIUM CARBONICUM	*In bed*
MENYANTHES	*With fever, migraine*
MERCURIUS SOLUBILIS	*With shaking, paralysis*
MYGALE	*Face and neck*
NUX VOMICA	
OPIUM	*Convulsions*
PHOSPHORUS	*Paralyzed areas*
PHYSOSTIGMA	*Eyelids*
PLATINA	
PLUMBUM	*With amyotrophy, paralysis*
STRAMONIUM	
STRYCHNINUM	
TARENTULA HISPANA	
THUYA (THUJA OCCIDENTALIS)	
VERATRUM VIRIDE	*Bouts of hypertension*
ZINCUM METALLICUM	*With restlessness of the lower limbs*

SHORTENING of tendons

See **TENDONS being too short**

SIGH (Need to)

See INHALE need to inhale

SLEEPINESS

FEVER and agitation (With)

PYROGENIUM
RHUS TOXICODENDRON

FEVER and prostration (With): *Adynamic febrile Syndrome*

ANTIMONIUM TARTARICUM *With paleness and weakness*
ARNICA
BAPTISIA
GELSEMIUM

FEVER (Without)

ANTIMONIUM TARTARICUM	
ARNICA	
CONIUM	
GELSEMIUM	
HELLEBORUS NIGER	
KALIUM CARBONICUM	*While eating*
NAJA NAJA (NAJA TRIPUDIANS)	
NUX MOSCHATA	*Permanent and insuperable*
OPIUM	
PHOSPHORICUM ACIDUM	

SORE MUSCLES

See also BRUISING

FEVER (With)

ARNICA	*Prostration, bed seems too hard*
BAPTISIA	*Prostration or agitation with hallucinations*
EUPATORIUM PERFORATUM	*Bones*
GELSEMIUM	*Great prostration*
PHYTOLACCA	*In the joints, aggravated by movement*
PYROGENIUM	*Infectious febrile syndrome*
RHUS TOXICODENDRON	

MUSCULAR OVEREXERTION (By)

ARNICA	*Continuous effort*
BELLIS PERENNIS	*Abdominal and pelvic muscles*
RHUS TOXICODENDRON	*Improved by slow movement*
RUTA GRAVEOLENS	*Violent effort*
SARCOLACTICUM ACIDUM	*At the slightest movement*

SPACING OF THE PELVIC BONES

MUREX	*Of the pubic symphysis during pregnancy, improved when patients' legs are crossed*
TRILLIUM PENDULUM	*Dysmenorrhea with sensation of hip and sacroiliac symphysis, improved by a tight bandage*

SPASM

See **CRAMPS**

SPIDER WEB on face

See **TENSION**

SPLINTER of wood (Splinter-like pain)

See also **STINGING PAIN**

AESCULUS HIPPOCASTANUM	*Anus*
AGARICUS MUSCARIUS	
ALUMINA	*Throat*
ARGENTUM NITRICUM	*ENT mostly*
HEPAR SULFUR	*With any inflammatory condition*
KALIUM CARBONICUM	*Throat*
NATRUM MURIATICUM	*Throat, anus*
NITRICUM ACIDUM	
PAEONIA	*Anus*
RATANHIA	*Anus*
SILICEA	*Often with an inflammatory condition*

SPLIT IN TWO

ANACARDIUM ORIENTALE	*Feels separated from the crowd; dual personality, two opposite wills are battling, during addictive behaviors for example*
BAPTISIA	*With feverish delirium, thinks the body is fragmented*
STRAMONIUM	*With fever, night terrors*

STABBING PAIN

See **THROBBING PAIN**

STEAM Hot coming out of the pores (At night)

FLUORICUM ACIDUM

STIFFNESS

IN THE JOINTS

ANGUSTURA	*Knees*
CALCAREA CARBONICA	*Arthritis with osteophytes, exostosis*
CALCAREA FLUORICA	*Arthritis with osteophytes, laxity*
CAUSTICUM	*Stiffness turning into ankylosis*
MEDORRHINUM	*Pelvic rheumatoid spondylitis*
NATRUM SULFURICUM	*Hip and knees*
RADIUM BROMATUM	*Spine*
RHUS TOXICODENDRON	*Improved by movement, with painful warming-up*
RUTA GRAVEOLENS	*Tendinous and periosteum trauma*
SULFUR (SULPHUR)	
TUBERCULINUM RESIDUUM	*Stiffness turning into ankylosis*

MUSCULAR

See also TENDONS too short

ACONITUM	*Pain in the nape of the neck, after a cold*
ACTAEA RACEMOSA (CIMICIFUGA)	*Para-vertebral chest area*
ANGUSTURA	*Muscle contracture and extensor cramps*
CAUSTICUM	*Torticolis*
GUAIACUM	*Gout*
LACHNANTES	*Torticolis*
NATRUM MURIATICUM	*Tendinous retraction*
PLUMBUM	*Paralysis of the extensors*
RUTA GRAVEOLENS	*Flexors*
STRYCHNINUM	
SULFUR (SULPHUR)	

STINGING PAIN

See THROBBING PAIN and also THORN

STOOLS

DONE (Sensation of defecation never being done)

MERCURIUS SOLUBILIS *Diarrhea*

IMPERIOUS in the morning

Gets subject out of bed

ALOE
LILIUM TIGRINUM
RUMEX
SULFUR (SULPHUR)

Upon waking up

BRYONIA

After breakfast

NATRUM SULFURICUM

In the morning

PODOPHYLLUM

INCOMPLETE

See FALSE URGES

RECTUM (In the)

GRAPHITES
LACHESIS MUTUS
OPIUM
SEPIA

STRETCH (Need to)

ANGUSTURA — *Relieves joint stiffness*
NITRICUM ACIDUM
RADIUM BROMATUM
THUYA (THUJA OCCIDENTALIS)
ZINCUM METALLICUM

STUFFED (Nose)

See OBSTRUCTION

SWARMING "Like insects crawling on skin"

See TINGLING

SWELLING (Of), Volume augmentation

BOVISTA
CHINA (CINCHONA)
NATRUM SULFURICUM
PLATINA — *Feels larger than it is in reality. Obsession with inexistent obesity [Guermonprez]*

EYES (Of the)

ACONITUM
ALUMINA
CHINA (CINCHONA)
COMOCLADIA DENTATA — *With tense throbbing pain*
PARIS QUADRIFOLIA
SPIGELIA ANTHELMIA

HANDS and FOREARMS (Of the)

ARANEA DIADEMA
BOVISTA

HEAD (Of the)

APIS
ARGENTUM NITRICUM — *Larger in volume, improved by a bandage and cold air*

BERBERIS	
BOVISTA	*Huge with headache, aggravation when putting something tight around it*
CROTALUS HORRIDUS	
GLONOINUM	*Pulsating, improved by a cold wrap*
NUX MOSCHATA	*Without headache*
PTELEA	*With a need to snack*

HEAD and the LIMBS (Of the)

BAPTISIA	
BOVISTA	
NUX MOSCHATA	
STRAMONIUM	*Feverish delirium*

HEART (Of the)

CENCHRIS	*Sensation of distended heart filling up the chest*
SPONGIA	
SULFUR (SULPHUR)	

OVARY (Of the left)

PLATINA

OVARY (Of the right)

PALLADIUM

TASTE

ACID

ARGENTUM NITRICUM	
CALCAREA CARBONICA	
LYCOPODIUM	
MAGNESIA CARBONICA	
NUX VOMICA	
PHOSPHORUS	*After drinking milk*

BITTER

ACONITUM	*Everything except water*
ARSENICUM ALBUM	
BRYONIA	
CHELIDONIUM	*Saliva*
CHINA (CINCHONA)	*Everything, including water*
HYDRASTIS	
KREOSOTUM	*Water*
MERCURIUS SOLUBILIS	
NATRUM MURIATICUM	
NATRUM SULFURICUM	

Sensations

NUX VOMICA	
PHOSPHORUS	*After eating*
PTELEA	
PULSATILLA	*Bread*
SULFUR (SULPHUR)	

BLOOD (Of)

ELAPS CORALLINUS	*Before coughing*

FETID (Of saliva)

MERCURIUS SOLUBILIS
NITRICUM ACIDUM

METALLIC

ARGENTUM NITRICUM
COCCULUS
CUPRUM METALLICUM
KALIUM BICHROMICUM
MERCURIUS SOLUBILIS

SALTY

CARBO VEGETABILIS	
CHINA (CINCHONA)	
MERCURIUS SOLUBILIS	
PHOSPHORUS	*Expectoration*
PULSATILLA	
SEPIA	
SULFUR (SULPHUR)	

Saliva (Of)

CYCLAMEN
NATRUM MURIATICUM
PHOSPHORUS

SWEET

MERCURIUS SOLUBILIS	
PULSATILLA	*Saliva*
SABADILLA	
STANNUM METALLICUM	
SULFUR (SULPHUR)	*Expectoration*

TEARING of the ANUS when defecating and hours after

NITRICUM ACIDUM	*Anal fissure*

TEARING of the LARYNX like a hook

ALLIUM CEPA	*With every cough*

TEETH

PULLED OUT

PRUNUS SPINOSA	*Facial neuralgia*

TOO LONG

HEPAR SULFUR	
LACHESIS MUTUS	
MAGNESIA CARBONICA	*Concomitant to dental neuralgia*
MEZEREUM	

TOO LONG AND LOOSE

MERCURIUS SOLUBILIS

TENDONS too short

AMMONIUM MURIATICUM	*Back side of the thigh*
ANGUSTURA	
CAUSTICUM	*Associated with overall stiffness*
COLOCYNTHIS	
DIOSCOREA	
GRAPHITES	*Achilles' tendon*
GUAIACUM	
MANGANUM	
NATRUM CARBONICUM	
NATRUM MURIATICUM	
PULSATILLA	
RUTA GRAVEOLENS	

TENESMUS (Anal, bladder)

See **FALSE painful URGE**

TENSION

BREASTS before menstruation

ASTERIAS RUBENS	*Left breast pulled inwards towards the center*
CALCAREA CARBONICA	
CONIUM	*Mastitis*
FOLLICULINUM	
GRAPHITES	
HELONIAS DIOICA	
MUREX	
NATRUM MURIATICUM	
PHYTOLACCA	*Mastitis*
PULSATILLA	
SEPIA	

Improved by wearing a bra, worsened by jolts

BRYONIA
LAC CANINUM

With intolerance to wearing a bra

LACHESIS MUTUS

SKIN of the face (Sensation of spider web on face)

ALUMINA	
BARYTA CARBONICA	
BORAX	
BROMUM	
GRAPHITES	*Forehead*
PETROLEUM	*Forehead*
SULFURICUM ACIDUM (SULPHURICUM ACIDUM)	*Coagulated egg white*

THIRST

In general

ACONITUM	
APIS	*During feverish shivering only*
ARNICA	*During feverish shivering only*
ARSENICUM ALBUM	
BELLADONNA	*Lemonade*
BRYONIA	
CHAMOMILLA	*With pain*
CHINA (CINCHONA)	
CINA	*With voracious hunger*
EUPATORIUM PERFOLIATUM	*Before vomiting*
IODUM	*With hunger*
MAGNESIA MURIATICA	*During headache*
MERCURIUS CORROSIVUS	
MERCURIUS SOLUBILIS	*In spite of moistened mouth*
NATRUM MURIATICUM	
PHOSPHORUS	
PYROGENIUM	*With fever*
RHUS TOXICODENDRON	
STRAMONIUM	*With fever*
SULFUR (SULPHUR)	*Drinks much and eats little*
VERATRUM ALBUM	

COLD DRINKS

ACONITUM
ARSENICUM ALBUM
BRYONIA
CHAMOMILLA
CHINA (CINCHONA)
CINA

EUPATORIUM PERFOLIATUM
MERCURIUS CORROSIVUS
MERCURIUS SOLUBILIS
NATRUM SULFURICUM
PHOSPHORUS
SILICEA
VERATRUM ALBUM *Ice cream*

DRYNESS of the mouth and the mucous membranes (With)

ALUMINA
ARNICA
BELLADONNA
BRYONIA
NATRUM MURIATICUM
STRAMONIUM

HYPERTHYROIDISM (With)

NATRUM MURIATICUM
SPONGIA

LARGE quantities (Intense drinking of)

With fever

ACONITUM
BRYONIA
EUPATORIUM PERFOLIATUM *Before vomiting*
MERCURIUS SOLUBILIS *In spite of wet mouth*
PHOSPHORUS
RHUS TOXICODENDRON

Without fever

NATRUM MURIATICUM
PHOSPHORUS
SULFUR (SULPHUR)
VERATRUM ALBUM

MILK Cold (For)

PHOSPHORUS
RHUS TOXICODENDRON
TUBERCULINUM

SMALL quantities (Intense drinking of)

ARSENICUM ALBUM
BELLADONNA *Little because of dysphagia and mainly because of dryness of the mouth*
CHINA (CINCHONA)
LACHESIS MUTUS *Cold water in acute diseases*
RHUS TOXICODENDRON
STRAMONIUM *With dysphagia*

Sensations

SULFUR (SULPHUR)

SWEAT (With)

CHINA (CINCHONA)	*Fever*

THORN

See **SPLINTER**

THROBBING PAIN, Pulsating, acute, stinging, stabbing

See also **SPLINTER**

AESCULUS HIPPOCASTANUM	*Hemorrhoids*
AGARICUS MUSCARIUS	*Like ice needles*
APIS	*And burning*
BERBERIS	*Renal colic or gallstones*
BORAX	*Chest pain*
BRYONIA	*Aggravated at the slightest movement*
CALCAREA CARBONICA	*Renal colic or gallstones*
CANTHARIS	*Pleural or colic pain*
CHELIDONIUM	*Renal colic*
COLLINSONIA	*Hemorrhoids*
CONIUM	*Along the nerve paths, with numbness*
DIOSCOREA	*Neuralgia*
KALIUM CARBONICUM	*Independent of movement, lower right area, chest*
KALIUM IODATUM	*Neuralgia or pain in the joints*
KALMIA	*Neuralgia*
LEDUM PALUSTRE	*Pain in the joints*
MERCURIUS SOLUBILIS	*Throat, hepatic area, base of the right lung*
NATRUM MURIATICUM	*Sacral-lumbar pain, anal fissure*
NATRUM SULFURICUM	*Hepatic area, left base of the lung*
NUX VOMICA	*With shaking*
OXALICUM ACIDUM	*Base of the left lung, with oxalic lithiasis*
PHELLANDRIUM	*From the right nipple towards the back between the shoulder blades*
PHYTOLACCA	*"Pins and needles"*
PLUMBUM	*Neuralgic pain of the spine or the limbs*
SULFUR (SULPHUR)	*Top of the left lung*
TABACUM	*Retro-sternal stabbing pain in the middle of the shoulder blade*
THUYA (THUJA OCCIDENTALIS)	*With myoclonus*

EAR (Near the)

CAPSICUM	*With mastoiditis painful to the touch*
MANGANUM	*All head pain is concentrated in the ears*

FACE (Near the): *Facial neuralgia*

ACONITUM	
AGARICUS MUSCARIUS	
ARSENICUM ALBUM	
BELLADONNA	
CAUSTICUM	
CEDRON	
CHAMOMILLA	
CHINA (CINCHONA)	
CHININUM SULFURICUM	
COLCHICUM	
COLOCYNTHIS	
LACHESIS MUTUS	
LYCOPODIUM	
MERCURIUS SOLUBILIS	
MEZEREUM	
NUX VOMICA	
PARIS QUADRIFOLIA	
PHOSPHORUS	
PLATINA	
PLUMBUM	
PRUNUS SPINOSA	*Eyes*
PULSATILLA	*With eye-watering*
SPIGELIA ANTHELMIA	*With eye-watering*
STANNUM METALLICUM	
THUYA (THUJA OCCIDENTALIS)	
VERBASCUM	

With sensation of cold

AGARICUS MUSCARIUS	*Like frostbite*
COLCHICUM	*Like frostbite*
LYCOPODIUM	
PLATINA	
THUYA (THUJA OCCIDENTALIS)	

INTERCOSTAL

ACTAEA RACEMOSA (CIMICIFUGA)	*Under the left breast*
ASCLEPIAS TUBEROSA	*Left*
DROSERA	*With spasmodic cough*
RANUNCULUS BULBOSUS	*From the liver to the right shoulder*
RUMEX	*Left lung, under the nipple, due to coughing*
SCILLA (SCILLA MARITIMA)	*Left pleurodynia*

NERVE PATHS (Along the)

COLOCYNTHIS	*Facial, sciatica*
HYPERICUM	*Centripetal direction*
KALMIA	*Centrifuge*
LACHNANTES	*Cervical-dorsal*

MAGNESIA CARBONICA	*Cervical-brachial neuralgia, nighttime causing patient to rise*
MAGNESIA PHOSPHORICA	
PLUMBUM	
THALLIUM ACETICUM	*Lower limbs*
THUYA (THUJA OCCIDENTALIS)	

TICKLING

See also **PRURITUS**

LARYNX (Of the), Like a feather

COCCUS CACTI	*In the late evening and when waking up*
DROSERA	*Aggravation due to the heat of the bed*

NOTCH (Of the) Substernal, leading to coughing

CHAMOMILLA
RUMEX

TRACHEA (Of the), Retro-sternal

AGARICUS MUSCARIUS	*Cough ending by sneezing*
CHINA (CINCHONA)	
IODUM	
STICTA PULMONARIA	

TIGHTNESS (Constriction, iron clamp, tight bandage)

ON MANY LEVELS

ANACARDIUM ORIENTALE	
CACTUS	
CAPSICUM	
COLOCYNTHIS	
LACHESIS MUTUS	*Key symptom of the medicine*

ANUS

CACTUS
LACHESIS MUTUS
LYCOPODIUM
NATRUM MURIATICUM
NUX VOMICA

CHEST

ACONITUM	*Sensation of being tied up*
ARGENTUM NITRICUM	*Aggravation when lying on the right side*
AURUM METALLICUM	*Aggravation when lying down; extrasystole*
CACTUS	*Sensation of being tied up, numbness of the left arm, aggravated when lying on the left side*
CROTALUS CASCAVELLA	

CUPRUM METALLICUM *Cyanosis*
HYDROCYANICUM ACIDUM *Cyanosis, esophageal spasm*
IODUM
LACHESIS MUTUS
LATRODECTUS MACTANS
LILIUM TIGRINUM *With numbness of the left arm*
LOBELIA *Asthma, vaso-vagal syndrome*
MOSCHUS *Choking sensation, of nervous origin*
NAJA NAJA (NAJA TRIPUDIANS) *With pain in the left arm*
NUX MOSCHATA
NUX VOMICA *Asthma, sensation of clothes being too tight*
PHOSPHORUS *Sensation of being tied up*
SPIGELIA ANTHELMIA *With palpitations, aggravated when lying on the left side*
TABACUM *Transfixing pain from the sternum to the back, paleness, aggravated when lying on the left side*

ESOPHAGUS

ZINCUM METALLICUM

HEAD (As if in tight helmet)

CACTUS
CARBO VEGETABILIS *With intolerance to wearing a hat*
CAUSTICUM
GELSEMIUM
GRAPHITES *Occiput*
IGNATIA
IODUM
MERCURIUS SOLUBILIS *Forehead*
NITRICUM ACIDUM
PHOSPHORICUM ACIDUM
SULFUR (SULPHUR)

HEART

ARSENICUM ALBUM
ARSENICUM IODATUM
LACHESIS MUTUS
NUX MOSCHATA

"Like grasped by a hand"

CACTUS
IODUM
LILIUM TIGRINUM

HYPOCHONDRIUM

ANACARDIUM ORIENTALE
DROSERA
IODUM

THROAT

BELLADONNA	*Dysphagia*
CENCHRIS	
CHAMOMILLA	*Asthma with sensation of a tightly-tied rope around the trachea*
CROTALUS HORRIDUS	
HYDROCYANICUM ACIDUM	
IGNATIA	
LACHESIS MUTUS	
LAUROCERASUS	
LYCOPUS	
NAJA NAJA (NAJA TRIPUDIANS)	
STRAMONIUM	

UTERUS

CACTUS
CHAMOMILLA
GELSEMIUM
NUX VOMICA
USTILAGO

TIME PASSING TOO SLOWLY

ALUMINA
AMBRA GRISEA
ARGENTUM NITRICUM
MEDORRHINUM
MERCURIUS SOLUBILIS

TINGLING

In general

AGARICUS MUSCARIUS	*Like insects crawling on skin*
CALCAREA PHOSPHORICA	
COLCHICUM	
HYPERICUM	
LYCOPODIUM	
NATRUM MURIATICUM	*On hyperventilation "terrain"*
NUX VOMICA	
PHOSPHORICUM ACIDUM	
PHOSPHORUS	
PLATINA	*On hyperventilation "terrain"*
RHUS TOXICODENDRON	
SECALE CORNUTUM	*Arteriopathy*
SULFUR (SULPHUR)	
ZINCUM METALLICUM	

EXTRIMITIES (Of the)

ACONITUM	*While writing*
AGARICUS MUSCARIUS	*On the surface of the skin and in the muscles*
AMMONIUM MURIATICUM	*Tip of fingers and toes*
COLCHICUM	*Under the fingernails*
GRAPHITES	*During menstruation*
KALMIA	*Left hand*
LYCOPODIUM	
NATRUM MURIATICUM	
NUX MOSCHATA	*Under the fingernails*
PHOSPHORUS	*With paralysis*
RHODODENDRON	
SECALE CORNUTUM	*Of vascular origin*
SILICEA	
THUYA (THUJA OCCIDENTALIS)	

Sensations

FOSSA NAVICULAR (Of the)

PETROSELINUM SATIVUM

"INSECTS (Like) Crawling on the skin"

ACONITUM	*Spine*
AGARICUS MUSCARIUS	

LIPS (Of the)

GELSEMIUM
MERCURIUS SOLUBILIS
NATRUM MURIATICUM

PAIN (With)

ACONITUM	
COLCHICUM	
THALLIUM ACETICUM	*Mostly to the extremities, of interest in the secondary iatrogenic effects of chemotherapy*

SOLES (Of the) of the feet

CAUSTICUM
COLOCYNTHIS

TINNITUS

See **BUZZING in the ears**

TRACTION

ABDOMEN towards the back

PLATINA

ANUS Upwards

PLUMBUM

BREAST Inwards

ASTERIAS RUBENS	*Left*
CROTON TIGLIUM	*During breastfeeding*

EYES Backwards

CROTON TIGLIUM
LACHESIS MUTUS
OLEANDER
PARIS QUADRIFOLIA
ZINCUM METALLICUM

UMBILICUS Backwards

With contracture of the abdominal muscles

PLUMBUM METALLICUM

URGE

STOOL (Urgent to go to the)

ALOE	*After eating, if urinating, passing gas*
ARGENTUM NITRICUM	*When anxious. Right after eating or drinking*
BERBERIS	*Constant urge*
COLOCYNTHIS	*After eating*
GELSEMIUM	*Anxiety*
LILIUM TIGRINUM	
MERCURIUS CORROSIVUS	
MERCURIUS SOLUBILIS	
RUMEX	*5 a.m.*
SULFUR (SULPHUR)	*When waking up, needs to get out of bed*

STOOL (Frequent urge to go to the), To no avail

See **FALSE URGES**

URINATE (Frequent urge to): *Pollakiuria*

ARGENTUM NITRICUM	
BARYTA CARBONICA	*Prostatism*
CANTHARIS	*With tenesmus*
CONIUM	*Prostatism*
DIGITALIS	
DULCAMARA	*As soon as subject gets cold*
GELSEMIUM	*Headaches improved by urinating with clear urine*
GRAPHITES	
IGNATIA	

LACHESIS MUTUS	*With tenesmus*
LYCOPODIUM	
MERCURIUS CORROSIVUS	*With tenesmus*
MERCURIUS SOLUBILIS	*With tenesmus*
NUX VOMICA	*With false urges*
OXALICUM ACIDUM	*As soon as subject thinks about it*
PAREIRA BRAVA	*With dysuria*
PHOSPHORICUM ACIDUM	*Clear urine*
PULSATILLA	*Lying on the back*
STAPHYSAGRIA	*Intense pain that stops when urinating*
SULFUR (SULPHUR)	
THUYA (THUJA OCCIDENTALIS)	*With pain*
VIBURNUM OPULUS	*With nausea and dysmenorrhea irradiating towards the front of the thighs*

VOMIT (To)

See NAUSEA

UTERUS (Feeling the)

HELONIAS DIOICA	
MUREX	*Painful sensation*

UVULA too long

COCCUS CACTI	*Sensation of a hair, bread crumb stuck in the throat*

VARIABLE

APPETITE

CINA
IGNATIA

MOOD

AMBRA GRISEA
COFFEA TOSTA
CROCUS SATIVUS
IGNATIA
MOSCHUS
NATRUM MURIATICUM
PLATINA
PULSATILLA
SUMBUL
VALERIANA

SENSATIONS Painful, in their localization and their nature

AMBRA GRISEA
MOSCHUS

PULSATILLA
TUBERCULINUM

VERTIGO

See DIZZINESS

VOLUME AUGMENTATION

See SWELLING

WADDLING GAIT

See DIZZINESS

WALK Unstable

See DIZZINESS

WATER Cold

POURED ON THE BODY

RHUS TOXICODENDRON

RUNNING THROUGH THE ENTIRE BODY

VERATRUM ALBUM

WEAKNESS

GENERAL

AMMONIUM CARBONICUM	*With hypersomnia and obsessing in daytime*
ANACARDIUM ORIENTALE	*Intellectual*
ARSENICUM ALBUM	*Out of proportion with the acute condition*
CALCAREA CARBONICA	*Fatigue, lack of endurance*
CARBO ANIMALIS	*Very altered general condition*
CARBO VEGETABILIS	*Extreme need to be fanned*
CAUSTICUM	
CHINA (CINCHONA)	*Following loss of fluids or fever*
COCCULUS	*After intellectual strain, staying up or working very late*
CONIUM	*After bowel movements*
GELSEMIUM	*General lassitude, with dozing off*
HYDRASTIS	*With alteration of the general state*
KALIUM CARBONICUM	*Muscular and cardiac at the slightest effort, with irritability. Exhausted after intercourse*
KALIUM PHOSPHORICUM	*Intellectual and sexual asthenia*
MANGANUM	*Great weakness. Obsessive need to lie down*
MERCURIUS CYANATUS	*Extreme weakness*
MERCURIUS SOLUBILIS	*Following infectious states*
MURIATICUM ACIDUM	*Physical then mental*

NATRUM MURIATICUM	*Following loss of fluids. Fatigue. Psychasthenia*
PHOSPHORICUM ACIDUM	*Mental then global*
PHOSPHORUS	*Alternating with excitement*
PICRICUM ACIDUM	*Great physical and mental lassitude. Obsessive need to lie down*
PODOPHYLLUM	*After bowel movement*
PSORINUM	*General physical and mental weakness, intensity close to ARSENICUM ALBUM*
SELENIUM	*Due to overexertion, excess or senescence. Obsessive need to lie down*
SEPIA	*Improved during menstruation*
SILICEA	*Lack of energy, vitality, obsessive need to lie down*
STANNUM METALLICUM	*Talking becomes difficult*
STAPHYSAGRIA	
ZINCUM METALLICUM	*Nervous, aggravated when talking*

LOCALIZED

CHEST, Unable to talk

DIGITALIS
PHOSPHORUS
STANNUM METALLICUM
SULFUR (SULPHUR)

FINGERS AND HANDS

CURARE — *Pianists*

KNEES

CAUSTICUM	
COBALTUM METALLICUM	*With sacrolumbar pain*
COCCULUS	*Sensation of knees giving out*
KALIUM CARBONICUM	*Sensation of knees giving out*
NUX MOSCHATA	
STAPHYSAGRIA	

LOWER LIMBS

ARGENTUM NITRICUM
CONIUM
GELSEMIUM

LUMBAR AREA

BERBERIS
CARBONEUM SULFURATUM
COCCULUS
KALIUM CARBONICUM

LUMBAR AREA AND KNEES

CAUSTICUM
COCCULUS
KALIUM CARBONICUM
OXALICUM ACIDUM
RADIUM BROMATUM

NECK

ABROTANUM
COCCULUS — *With sensation that head is too heavy to lift*

Sensations

INTELLECTUAL OVEREXERTION (Weakness after)

ANACARDIUM ORIENTALE	*Extensive memory loss*
FLUORICUM ACIDUM	*Alternating hypomanic phases with great physical activity*
KALIUM PHOSPHORICUM	*Headaches, insomnia, memory loss, sexual asthenia*
NATRUM MURIATICUM	*Often leads to giving up or failing*
PHOSPHORICUM ACIDUM	*Headaches. Memory loss. Depression*
SILICEA	*Attention and memory deficiency, little capacity to work, easily tired*

SIGHT, Eye strain (Accommodation)

AGARICUS MUSCARIUS	*Elderly people*
ARGENTUM NITRICUM	
AURUM METALLICUM	*Enlarged congested and painful eyes. Glaucoma frequent*
CINA	
COCCULUS	
CONIUM	
GELSEMIUM	
MANGANUM	
NATRUM MURIATICUM	*Eye pain when reading*
ONOSMODIUM	
PHYSOSTIGMA	*Following visual strain*
RADIUM BROMATUM	
RUTA GRAVEOLENS	*Painful, following visual strain*
SENEGA	*Vertical diplopia*

WEIGHT

ANUS (Near the)

ALOE

HEAD (Around the)

CARBO VEGETABILIS	
COCCULUS	
GELSEMIUM	
GLONOINUM	
NAJA NAJA (NAJA TRIPUDIANS)	
NUX MOSCHATA	*With sleepiness and dizziness*
ZINCUM METALLICUM	

PELVIS (Near the level of the): *Bearing down*

CARBO VEGETABILIS
HELONIAS DIOICA
LAC CANINUM

LILIUM TIGRINUM	*Sensation that the urogenital organs are going to drop through the vulva*
MUREX	
NATRUM CARBONICUM	
NATRUM MURIATICUM	*In the morning*
PALLADIUM	*With pain in the right ovary*
PLATINA	
SEPIA	*With painful lumbar irradiation*
VIBURNUM OPULUS	*With pain irradiating to the front of the thighs*

With sexual arousal

LILIUM TIGRINUM
MUREX

STERNUM (Crushing around the)

ARSENICUM ALBUM
AURUM METALLICUM
NAJA NAJA (NAJA TRIPUDIANS)
PHOSPHORUS

STOMACH (On the level of the): *Sensation of stones in the stomach*

BRYONIA
CHAMOMILLA
KALIUM BICHROMICUM
NUX VOMICA
PULSATILLA

Far from meals

LYCOPODIUM
NUX VOMICA

VERTEX (Near the)

CACTUS
GLONOINUM
LACHESIS MUTUS
MENYANTHES
PHOSPHORICUM ACIDUM
ZINCUM METALLICUM

WELL-BEING Exceptional

The day before onset of disease

PSORINUM	*Migraine*

WET (Of being)

BACK (Clothes touching the) is wet

TUBERCULINUM

WET STOCKINGS

CALCAREA CARBONICA
SEPIA

WOUND Open, GRAZE

GENITO-URINARY MUCOUS MEMBRANES (Around the)

CANTHARIS
CAUSTICUM
NITRICUM ACIDUM

LARYNX (Near the)

ACONITUM
ALLIUM CEPA *By coughing*
ARGENTUM METALLICUM
ARUM TRIPHYLLUM
BROMUM
CAUSTICUM
DROSERA
NITRICUM ACIDUM
PHOSPHORUS
RUMEX
SPONGIA

SOFT PALATE (Around the)

AMBRA GRISEA

TRACHEA (Around the)

RUMEX
SANGUINARIA CANADENSIS

DISCHARGES AND MENSTRUATION

Discharges are physiological fluids elaborated by the glandular epithelia. Except for **lactation**, these fluids are continually secreted in varying amounts as the body needs them.

Discharges help maintain the equilibrium of the body:
- for some, by their HORMONAL ACTION,
- for others, by their ENZYMATIC ACTION as is the case for saliva.

They ensure a PROTECTIVE MECHANICAL ROLE against outside aggressions (lachrymal discharge).

Discharges can be:
- either EXOCRINE and, as such, are evacuated by excretory channels towards the outside or towards another organ,
- or ENDOCRINE, which means that they are evacuated directly into the blood.

Only **physiological discharges** that are MODIFIED IN QUANTITY AND QUALITY are taken into account. Integrated into a general nosological context, they can help for choosing the right homeopathic medicine.

The aspect and quantity of **saliva** serve to complete clinical descriptions and are only secondary symptoms.

Sweat is generally easily observable and accurately described by patients. This is a particular symptom that is part of the general objective symptoms. It is always important to consider perspiration in order to determine the appropriate medicine, both for acute and chronic problems.
- In acute feverish conditions, observation of the onset, localization, odor, quantity and timing of sweat is essential in choosing the right medicine;
- In chronic cases, the study of sweat helps indicate medicines of general action, for which perspiration is a general sign of much value (for example, the fetid odor of foot sweat in SILICEA).

Menstrual periods are not actually discharges, but rather a physiological syndrome characterized by periodic blood flow (menstruation), due to the elimination of uterine mucous membranes (occurring in women when there is no fecundation, from puberty to menopause).

The following have been excluded from this chapter:
- discharges such as stools, urine, breath, etc.
- bleeding/hemorrhaging

This chapter will be divided as follows:

I - MUCOUS MEMBRANE DISCHARGES

ABSENCE (Dryness of the mucous membranes)

ACONITUM	*Dryness of the skin and mucous membranes at the beginning of acute feverish conditions*
ALUMINA	*Dryness of the skin and mucous membranes, in a chronic condition, constipation*
BELLADONNA	*Inflammatory symptoms of the mucous membranes, with fever; dryness of the mucous membranes contrasting with the moistness of the skin in feverish conditions*
BRYONIA	*Dryness of all mucous membranes, with intense thirst for large quantities, at long intervals*
KALIUM BICHROMICUM	*Beginning of a cold with sensation of plugged-up nose and pressure at the base of the nose*
LYCOPODIUM	*Vaginal dryness, with dry skin*
NATRUM MURIATICUM	*Dryness of the mucous membranes alternating with flowing conditions*
NUX MOSCHATA	*Dryness of all mucous membranes: dry mouth with no thirst with abdominal bloating, constipation; dry eyes*
NUX VOMICA	*At the beginning of respiratory and ENT disorders*
OPIUM	*Diminution of all discharges, except sweat and breast milk*
PULSATILLA	*Dryness of the mucous membranes with no thirst*
SAMBUCUS	*Dry and plugged-up nose*
SANGUINARIA CANADENSIS	*Dry and burning mucous membranes that fissure or excoriate; digestive and respiratory polarities*
SEPIA	*Vaginal dryness*
STICTA PULMONARIA	*Dry cough, nasal obstruction with inefficient urge to blow ones nose*
SULFUR (SULPHUR)	*Burning dryness improved by cold*

ABUNDANT

ALLIUM CEPA	*Irritant nasal discharge, improved by fresh air, with non-irritant eye-watering*
ALUMINA	*Abundant and irritant leukorrhea*
AMMONIUM MURIATICUM	*Irritant nasal discharge with anosmia and sensation of plugged-up nose*
ANTIMONIUM TARTARICUM	*Lung obstruction sometimes with fluttering of the nostrils*
ARALIA RACEMOSA	*Rhinitis with watery irritant discharge and sneezing aggravated by drafts; cough and asthma aggravated at bedtime*
ARSENICUM ALBUM	*Burning, irritant discharge with improvement by heat on a general and local condition*

Remedy	Indication
COCCUS CACTI	*Thread-like mucus with whooping cough aggravated before midnight and in the morning when waking up*
EUPHRASIA	*Burning eye-watering improved by heat, with non-irritant catarrh*
KALIUM BICHROMICUM	*Coryza first flowing and abundant, then becoming thick with sticky viscous discharges, greenish-yellow*
KALIUM IODATUM	*Watery flow, irritant with red and swollen nose, abundant then purulent; sensation of pressure at the base of the nose and pain in the sinuses; aggravation due to cold; associated ocular disorders with swollen, red watery eyes*
MERCURIUS SOLUBILIS	*Tendency to suppuration with greenish-yellow discharge*
NAPHTALINUM	*Abundant coryza, highly excoriating, improved with fresh air, with irritant eye-watering*
NATRUM MURIATICUM	*Catarrh and profuse eye-watering alternating with a dryness of the mucous membranes, irritant leukorrhea*
PHELLANDRIUM	*Chronic pulmonary suppuration, with abundant and highly fetid expectoration*
PHOSPHORUS	*Abundant watery catarrh alternating with dry nose, olfactory hypersensitivity; tendency to epistaxis*
PULSATILLA	*Mucopurulent discharge, non-irritant, except for leukorrhea at times*
SANGUINARIA CANADENSIS	*Flowing coryza, abundant, burning, excoriating in the nostrils, with sneezing, hypersensitivity to odors, mainly of flowers*
SENEGA	*Cough ending with sneezing, lung congestion with difficult expectoration*
SILICEA	*Indicated in chronic inflammation of the mucous membranes in sensitive-type patients*
THUYA (THUJA OCCIDENTALIS)	*During chronic conditions*

ACID

Remedy	Indication
IRIS VERSICOLOR	*Burning of all the digestive tube, from mouth to anus, with hypersalivation*
KALIUM BICHROMICUM	*Heartburn, pyrosis with tendency towards ulcers, aggravated by beer*
MAGNESIA CARBONICA	*Digestive hyper-acidity and pyrosis, with milk intolerance*
ROBINIA	*Nocturnal acid gastralgia*
SULFURICUM ACIDUM (SULPHURICUM ACIDUM)	*Gastric esophageal reflux, with burning in stomach and esophagus, mouth ulcers*

ALTERNATION of flowing and obstruction of the nose

Remedy	Indication
DULCAMARA	*Coryza with cervical adenopathy after exposure to damp cold*
HEPAR SULFUR	*Intense painful local phenomena*

HYDRASTIS	*Aggravation due to cold, except nasal obstruction aggravated by heat*
NATRUM MURIATICUM	*General characteristic for all mucous membranes*
NUX VOMICA	*Nasal obstruction at night and due to heat, catarrh in daytime*
PHOSPHORUS	*With a tendency to epistaxis; alternation of dryness and watery catarrh; olfactory hypersensitivity*

BLOODY

BRONCHIAL

ACONITUM	*Dryness and spasms, anxiety*
ARNICA	
BRYONIA	*Rusty sputum*
FERRUM PHOSPHORICUM	*Indicated in acute congestive conditions*
IPECA (IPECAC)	
KALIUM BICHROMICUM	
LACHESIS MUTUS	
PHOSPHORUS	*Prescribe with caution if history of tuberculosis*
SANGUINARIA CANADENSIS	*Expectoration sometimes blood-streaked*

DIGESTIVE

ARSENICUM ALBUM	*Thirsty for small quantities of cold water, vomited out once warmed in the stomach*
CHINA (CINCHONA)	*Associated abdominal bloating*
IPECA (IPECAC)	*Nausea and hypersalivation*
KALIUM BICHROMICUM	*Indicated in gastric pathologies or vomiting following a cough*
PHOSPHORUS	*Thirsty for large quantities of cold water, rapidly vomited*
MERCURIUS CORROSIVUS	*Extensive tenesmus*

ENT

ARGENTUM NITRICUM	*Dark red mucous membranes, splinter-like pain felt on the mucous membranes*
ARUM TRIPHYLLUM	
FERRUM PHOSPHORICUM	
GRAPHITES	
HEPAR SULFUR	*Greenish discharge sometimes streaked with blood*
HYDRASTIS	*Thick, viscous yellowish discharge*
IPECA (IPECAC)	
KALIUM BICHROMICUM	*Plugs and scabs in the nostrils*
KALIUM IODATUM	
KREOSOTUM	*Gums with a dark red or bluish lining, hypersalivation and fetid breath*
MERCURIUS SOLUBILIS	*Rhinopharyngitis, with sore throat and stomatitis*
MEZEREUM	*Irritant and excoriating coryza with malar pain*
PHOSPHORUS	*Tendency to epistaxis*

SULFURICUM ACIDUM (SULPHURICUM ACIDUM)	
	Ulceration and mouth ulcers with darkish bleeding

BRONCHIAL

ACONITUM	*Indicated at the onset of acute disorders occurring after cold; dry skin*
AMMONIUM CARBONICUM	*Bronchial congestion with difficult expectoration during cardiorespiratory decompensation*
ANTIMONIUM TARTARICUM	*Bronchial congestion with inefficient cough*
ARALIA RACEMOSA	*Asthma and coughing at the beginning of the night*
ARNICA	*Spasmodic coughing, painful, with crying before the cough in children*
ARSENICUM ALBUM	*Asthma or bronchitis with intense dyspnea, anxiety, aggravation between 1 and 3 a.m.*
ARSENICUM IODATUM	*Thick expectoration*
BELLADONNA	*Indicated at the onset of acute disorders occurring after cold; clammy skin*
BLATTA ORIENTALIS	*Bronchitis with asthma and bronchial congestion, without alteration of the general condition*
BROMUM	*Asthma improved at the seaside or at sea*
BRYONIA	*Dryness of the mucous membranes and exudation from the serous membranes*
CALCAREA SULPHURICA	*Abundant expectoration during inflammatory respiratory conditions; mostly chronic bronchitis*
CARBO VEGETABILIS	*Acute respiratory disorders with cyanosis, pain and alteration of the general condition*
CAUSTICUM	*Painful cough with dyspnea and urinary incontinence*
CHAMOMILLA	*Bronchitis in infants when teething*
DULCAMARA	*Disorders occurring in damp weather*
FERRUM PHOSPHORICUM	*Pulmonary congestive phenomena*
GRINDELIA	*Bronchial congestion, choking feeling when going to sleep and waking up*
HEPAR SULFUR	*Purulent expectoration*
HYDRASTIS	*Yellow, viscous and sticky expectoration*
HYPERICUM	*Asthma and disorders aggravated by dampness and fog*
IPECA (IPECAC)	*Whooping cough; asthma with sibilant sounds, pink and humid tongue, paleness and nausea*
KALIUM BICHROMICUM	*Yellow, viscous and sticky expectoration*
KALIUM CARBONICUM	*Disorders occurring sometimes in a context of cardiorespiratory insufficiency, dyspnea with difficult expectoration so subject sits down with elbows on knees; pain and congestion in the right base; sometimes edema in the internal angle of the upper eyelid*
KALIUM IODATUM	*Respiratory disorders aggravated at 3 a.m. with irritant ENT discharge*
KALIUM MURIATICUM	*Difficult viscous expectoration with ENT signs*
LYCOPODIUM	*Affection of the base of the right lung; sometimes dyspnea and fluttering of the nostrils; salty-tasting expectoration*

MERCURIUS SOLUBILIS	*Dry cough at night and loose in the day, with purulent expectoration*
NATRUM MURIATICUM	*Asthma with alternation of spasmodic and catarrh attacks; sometimes aggravated between 1 and 3 a.m.*
NATRUM SULFURICUM	*Loose productive cough, aggravated around 5 a.m., by damp weather, at the seaside; asthma, bronchitis or pneumonia of the left base; painful cough makes one compress the chest with both hands*
PHELLANDRIUM	*Abundant and very fetid expectoration*
PHOSPHORUS	*Tiring dry cough, hoarseness and laryngeal burns, worse in the evening*
PSORINUM	*Alternation of skin and respiratory disorders*
PULSATILLA	*Nocturnal dry cough and daytime loose cough, with yellow expectoration or changing color during the day*
SANGUINARIA CANADENSIS	*Expectoration, sometimes bloody*
SENEGA	*Cough with dyspnea preventing patient from lying down, cough ending with sneezing*
SEPIA	
SILICEA	*Chronic bronchial-pulmonary infections with suppuration, aggravated by cold, infections*
STANNUM METALLICUM	*Fetid expectoration sometimes containing small black clots, tiring cavernous cough with hoarseness*
SULFUR (SULPHUR)	*Alternating or concomitant cutaneous and respiratory disorders*
SULFUR IODATUM (SULPHUR IODATUM)	*Lingering cough after bronchitis*
THUYA (THUJA OCCIDENTALIS)	
TUBERCULINUM	

COLORLESS

See also **WATERY**

ALLIUM CEPA	*Watery discharge*
ANTIMONIUM TARTARICUM	
ARALIA RACEMOSA	
ARSENICUM ALBUM	
ARUM TRIPHYLLUM	
CALCAREA PHOSPHORICA	*"Egg-white" leukorrhea*
COCCUS CACTI	
CORALLIUM RUBRUM	*Face red; thick and thread-like mucus with posterior discharge*
EUPHRASIA	*Watery eyes and catarrh*
IPECA (IPECAC)	
KALIUM IODATUM	*At the beginning of rhinitis: watery, irritant and abundant discharge*
NATRUM MURIATICUM	*"Egg-white" leukorrhea*
NUX VOMICA	
PHOSPHORUS	
RUMEX CRISPUS	*Fear of inhaling cold air, with aggravation*
SABADILLA	

CONJUNCTIVA

ACONITUM	
ALLIUM CEPA	*Non-irritant discharge*
APIS	*Edema, dryness and redness*
ARGENTUM NITRICUM	*Splinter-like pain, photophobia and tendency towards ulceration*
ARSENICUM ALBUM	*Burning sensation improved by heat*
BELLADONNA	*Redness of the conjunctiva with photophobia, dryness or eye-watering*
EUPHRASIA	*Abundant and irritant eye-watering with photophobia*
GRAPHITES	*Photophobia, crusty and oozing lesions of the eyelids*
HEPAR SULFUR	*Local splinter-like sensation*
KALIUM BICHROMICUM	*Ulcerative tendency with thread-like discharge*
KALIUM IODATUM	*Irritant eye-watering and nasal discharge, conjunctivitis, aggravated by fresh air and wind*
MEDORRHINUM	*Notion of chronic infection of the urogenital area*
MERCURIUS CORROSIVUS	*Aggravation due to heat and photophobia*
MERCURIUS SOLUBILIS	*Discharge rapidly becomes mucopurulent*
NAPHTALINUM	*Spasmodic coryza with irritant nasal and ocular discharge*
PULSATILLA	*Lingering thick yellow discharge, styes*
SEPIA	*Aggravation at night and with fresh air*
STAPHYSAGRIA	*Styes*
SULFUR (SULPHUR)	*Important congestive phenomena; burning sensation*
THUYA (THUJA OCCIDENTALIS)	*Chronic and recurring infections; recurring styes*

CRUSTY

ALUMINA	*Due to dryness of the mucous membranes*
AMMONIUM CARBONICUM	*Nose plugged with scabs, mostly in newborns*
ELAPS	*Fetid ENT discharge*
GRAPHITES	*Scabs in nose*
KALIUM BICHROMICUM	*Thick mucus forming clots and yellowish crusts*
MEZEREUM	*Bloody crusts in the nasal cavity during chronic sinusitis and rhinitis*
SEPIA	*Crusts in the nose*
SULFUR (SULPHUR)	
THUYA (THUJA OCCIDENTALIS)	
TUBERCULINUM	*Crusts in the nose*

DRYNESS

See **ABSENCE**

EAR (Middle ear and eustachian tube)

ARSENICUM ALBUM	*Acute otitis, a systematic prescription for some*
ARSENICUM IODATUM	*Chronic serous otitis; allergic "terrain"*

AURUM METALLICUM	*Risks of mastoiditis suppuration, chronic otitis*
AVIAIRE	*Recurring otitis*
CAUSTICUM	*Recurring otitis in a sensitive-type child*
ELAPS	*Suppuration and fetid discharge*
FERRUM PHOSPHORICUM	*Pain and tympanic congestion*
GRAPHITES	*Medicine for external otitis with honey-like discharge*
HEPAR SULFUR	*Caution, if there is a risk of suppuration*
KALIUM MURIATICUM	*Acute or chronic rhinitis with eustachian tube catarrh*
KALIUM SULFURICUM	
LACHESIS MUTUS	*Painful otitis with risk of suppuration*
MANGANUM ACETICUM	*Chronic sero-mucous otitis, aggravated by dampness*
MERCURIUS DULCIS	*Mainly indicated in serous otitis with eustachian tube catarrh, doubtful efficacy*
MERCURIUS SOLUBILIS	
NATRUM MURIATICUM	*Chronic medicine in recurring problems*
PULSATILLA	
SILICEA	*Recurring and chronic otitis*
SULFUR (SULPHUR)	
TELLURIUM	*Excoriating chronic otorrhea*
TUBERCULINUM	*Recurring otitis ELAPS*

EXCORIATING

ARGENTUM NITRICUM	*Inflammation and ulceration of the mucous membranes*
ARSENICUM ALBUM	*Inflammation and ulceration of the mucous membranes*
ARSENICUM IODATUM	*Discharge more burning and excoriating than ARSENICUM ALBUM*
ARUM TRIPHYLLUM	*Bloody excoriation of the nostrils and upper lip*
BORAX	*Mouth ulcers*
FLUORICUM ACIDUM	*Ulceration with inflammatory peri-ulcerous reactions*
KALIUM BICHROMICUM	*Deep ulceration with regular cutter-like edges*
KREOSOTUM	*Ulceration and excoriation with bloody discharge*
MERCURIUS CORROSIVUS	*Inflammation of the mucous membranes with more pronounced pain, burning and tenesmus than MERCURIUS SOLUBILIS*
MERCURIUS SOLUBILIS	*Superficial infected ulceration*
NITRICUM ACIDUM	*Ulceration that bleeds easily, slit-like fissures*
SANGUINARIA CANADENSIS	*Flowing coryza, abundant burning, excoriating the nostrils, with sneezing, hypersensitivity to odors, mostly flowers*
SULFURICUM ACIDUM (SULPHURICUM ACIDUM)	*Burning ulceration with bloody and fetid discharge*
TELLURIUM	*Chronic and excoriating otorrhea*

FETID

AURUM METALLICUM	*Chronic inflammation of the nose, sinuses or ears*
BENZOICUM ACIDUM	*Dark urine smelling like horse urine. The odor impregnates clothes and body*
HEPAR SULFUR	*Acute tendency of the mucous membranes to suppuration*

KALIUM IODATUM	*Sinusitis with supra-orbital pain*
MERCURIUS SOLUBILIS	*Suppuration of the mucous membranes*
PSORINUM	*Foul odor of the skin and discharge*
SULFUR (SULPHUR)	*All discharges*

FILAMENTOUS

COCCUS CACTI	*Whooping cough bringing up filamentous mucus, face red and nausea when coughing; aggravation before midnight and when waking up*
CORALLIUM RUBRUM	*Explosive spasmodic cough with face red when coughing, rhinitis with filamentous post-nasal discharge, aggravation due to cold air*
HYDRASTIS	*Rhinitis with yellowish mucus streaked with blood, with posterior discharge*
KALIUM BICHROMICUM	*Formation of mucous bubbles mucus when nose is strongly blown; elastic yellowish plugs in the nasal cavity*

GENITAL mucous membranes

ALUMINA	*Profuse leukorrhea, white or yellowish, excoriating*
ARGENTUM NITRICUM	*With fetid and irritant ulceration*
ARSENICUM ALBUM	*Yellowish, putrid, fetid and corrosive leukorrhea, with burning improved by application of hot wraps*
BORAX	*Genital ulcers, herpes, "egg-white" discharge; tendency to ulcerate*
CALCAREA CARBONICA	*Milky leukorrhea*
CALCAREA PHOSPHORICA	*"Egg-white" leukorrhea*
FRAXINUS AMERICANA	*Abundant watery discharge in a context of uterine fibroid with sensation of ptosis*
GRAPHITES	*White, profuse and irritant leukorrhea, with pruritus*
HELONIAS DIOICA	*Characteristic leukorrhea looking like curdled milk, uterine ptosis sensation*
HEPAR SULFUR	*Greenish, very fetid leukorrhea with uterine and ovarian pain*
HYDRASTIS	*Yellowish, viscous and filamentous leukorrhea*
KALIUM BICHROMICUM	*Similar to HYDRASTIS with a tendency to ulceration with clean-cut borders that look they were made by cookie-cutters*
KREOSOTUM	*Genital ulceration*
MEDORRHINUM	*Chronic and recurring infections, fetid and/or briny odor*
MERCURIUS CORROSIVUS	*Leukorrhea similar to that of MERCURIUS SOLUBILIS but more acute and a more pronounced tendency to ulcerate*
MERCURIUS SOLUBILIS	*Irritant greenish-yellow leukorrhea with a tendency to ulceration on the cervix*
NATRUM MURIATICUM	*"Egg-white" leukorrhea alternating with bouts of dryness of the mucous membranes*
NITRICUM ACIDUM	*Cervix ulceration with splinter-like pain and bleeding at the slightest contact*

PULSATILLA	*Lingering leukorrhea outside of an infection, variable in aspect, little or not irritant*
SEPIA	*"Bearing-down" sensation; vesicles on the skin and the mucous membranes; white or yellowish leukorrhea, excoriating and burning*
SILICEA	*Chronic leukorrhea with a tendency towards vesicles and fistulas*
SULFUR (SULPHUR)	*Burning irritation with fetid discharge*
THUYA (THUJA OCCIDENTALIS)	*Chronic disorders*

GRAYISH

ARGENTUM METALLICUM	*Chronic pharyngitis or laryngitis with grayish mucus*
KALIUM CARBONICUM	*Night, asthma attacks between 2 and 4 a.m., with a need to sit up in bed, elbows on knees, attack ending with expectoration of tapioca-like sputum*
KALIUM MURIATICUM	*Nasal mucus and expectoration*
LYCOPODIUM	*During rhinitis and bronchitis*

GREENISH YELLOW

See also **MUCOPURULENT**

AURUM METALLICUM	
HEPAR SULFUR	
HYDRASTIS	*Viscous and filamentous mucus of all mucous membranes*
KALIUM BICHROMICUM	*Viscous and filamentous mucus of all mucous membranes, sometimes forming scabs and plugs in the nose*
KALIUM IODATUM	
KALIUM SULFURICUM	
MEDORRHINUM	
MERCURIUS SOLUBILIS	
NATRUM SULFURICUM	*Painful coughing with need to compress the thorax during the coughing spells*
PULSATILLA	*ENT and genital discharge, sometimes irritant*
SEPIA	
SILICEA	*Chronic infections*
SULFUR (SULPHUR)	
THUYA (THUJA OCCIDENTALIS)	

IRRITATING

ALLIUM CEPA	*Around the nose, and non-irritant at eye level*
AMMONIUM MURIATICUM	*Irritant nasal discharge with anosmia and sensation of stuffed nose*
ARALIA RACEMOSA	*Aggravation due to wind drafts, asthma aggravated at the beginning of the night and at bedtime*
ARUM TRIPHYLLUM	*Very irritant catarrh, with nostrils and upper lip*

	excoriated and bloody; voice timbre varies during laryngitis
ARSENICUM ALBUM	*Burning sensation improved by heat generally and locally*
ARSENICUM IODATUM	*Chronic affection of the mucous membranes, burning discharge, cold sensitivity less pronounced than ARSENICUM ALBUM*
BROMUM	*Watery and excoriating coryza; improved at the seaside and at sea; hoarse cough*
EUPHRASIA	*Of the eyes but not of the nose, improved by heat*
HEPAR SULFUR	*Oozing tendency with fetid discharge and intense pain*
KALIUM IODATUM	*Irritant conjunctiva and nasal discharge*
MERCURIUS CORROSIVUS	
MERCURIUS SOLUBILIS	*Oozing tendency*
NAPHTALINUM	*Affection of the nasal and ocular mucous membranes during acute or spasmodic coryza*
SABADILLA	*Watery discharge with irritant tears; need to rub the soft palate with the tongue*
SULFUR (SULPHUR)	

LARYNGEAL and TRACHEAL

ALLIUM CEPA	*Painful laryngeal cough with need to grasp the neck during the coughing spell*
ARGENTUM METALLICUM	*Sensation of an open larynx wound; hoarseness or aphonia for singers or public speakers; sometimes cough with rejection of viscous grayish mucus*
ARGENTUM NITRICUM	*Splinter-like sensation in the mucous membranes with continuous need to clear the throat and hoarseness; sometimes emotion-induced*
BROMUM	*Suffocating croup-like cough improved when drinking cold beverages, at seaside or at sea*
CAUSTICUM	*Hoarseness aggravated in the morning with sensation of open larynx wound, improved when drinking cold water*
COCCUS CACTI	*Laryngeal tickling leading to whooping-like cough, with aggravation around 11:30 p.m. and when waking up, improvement with cold air and drinking cold beverages*
CORALLIUM RUBRUM	*Spasmodic cough with facial congestion during coughing spells*
HEPAR SULFUR	*Hoarse choking cough, aggravation due to cold*
IODUM	
KALIUM IODATUM	*Aggravation in the second half of the night*
MANGANUM ACETICUM	*Hoarseness caused by damp cold or by prolonged talking; chronic laryngeal cough with hoarse voice and need to clear the throat in order to speak clearly*
RUMEX CRISPUS	*Dry cough provoked by inhaling cold air and pressure on the sub-sternal notch; accompanied by retro-sternal pruritus and urinary incontinence when coughing*

MUCOPURULENT, purulent

IN GENERAL

PYROGENIUM — *Prevention or stopping of any acute oozing condition*

SERUM DE YERSIN (SERUM: YERSIN) — *Prevention of bacterial over-infection*

BRONCHIAL

ARSENICUM IODATUM — *Thick expectoration*

CALCAREA SULFURICA — *Abundant expectoration during respiratory inflammatory conditions especially chronic bronchitis*

HEPAR SULFUR — *Difficult expectoration with choking*

HYDRASTIS

KALIUM BICHROMICUM

KREOSOTUM — *Highly fetid expectoration*

MERCURIUS SOLUBILIS

NATRUM SULFURICUM

PHELLANDRIUM — *Highly fetid expectoration*

PULSATILLA — *Chronic discharge, not excessively sticky*

SILICEA

STANNUM METALLICUM — *Fetid expectoration sometimes with little black clots, tiring cavernous cough, with hoarseness*

SULFUR IODATUM (SULPHUR IODATUM)

CONJUNCTIVA

ARGENTUM NITRICUM — *Ulcerative tendency*

HEPAR SULFUR — *Local splinter-like sensation*

MEDORRHINUM — *Previous urogenital infections*

MERCURIUS SOLUBILIS — *Aggravation due to heat and photophobia*

PULSATILLA — *Lingering thick yellow discharge; styes*

SULFUR (SULPHUR) — *Extensive congestive phenomena; burning sensation*

THUYA (THUJA OCCIDENTALIS) — *Chronic and recurring infections; recurring styes*

DIGESTIVE

ARGENTUM NITRICUM — *Dysenteric syndrome*

ARSENICUM ALBUM — *Dysenteric syndrome*

MERCURIUS CORROSIVUS — *Mucopurulent stools more bloody and painful than MERCURIUS SOLUBILIS*

MERCURIUS SOLUBILIS — *Dysenteric syndrome*

ENT

ARSENICUM ALBUM — *Dental abscess*

AURUM METALLICUM — *Chronic rhinitis often with associated chronic sinusitis*

CINNABARIS (MERCURIUS SULPHURATUS RUBER) — *Posterior catarrh with filamentous mucus; pain on the ridge of the nose with localization sometimes around the eye-sockets; the eye is bright red*

HEKLA LAVA	*Oozing of the gums*
HEPAR SULFUR	*Pain and oozing of the affected mucous membranes*
HYDRASTIS	*Thick, viscous and very sticky discharge, yellowish, with flow into the nasal part of pharynx*
KALIUM BICHROMICUM	*Discharge like those of HYDRASTIS, with sensation of pressure at the base of the nose*
KALIUM IODATUM	*Sometimes fetid flow*
LACHESIS MUTUS	*Mucous membranes grow darker with intense dysphagia and risk of left tonsil abscess; sometimes blocked sinusitis*
LYCOPODIUM	
MERCURIUS CYANATUS	*Pultaceous sore throat*
MERCURIUS SOLUBILIS	*Purulent, greenish, abundant discharge, excoriating the nostrils*
MEZEREUM	*Burning pain in the nose and face bones, mucopurulent catarrh streaked with blood*
NATRUM SULFURICUM	*Greenish discharge, and posterior blowing in chronic rhinopharyngitis*
PULSATILLA	*Thick, non-irritant discharge; frequent anosmia*
SILICEA	
SULFUR (SULPHUR)	
SULFUR IODATUM (SULPHUR IODATUM)	*Recurring ENT pathologies with cervical adenopathy*
THUYA (THUJA OCCIDENTALIS)	

GENITAL

HEPAR SULFUR	*Purulent and foul-smelling leukorrhea with uterine and ovarian pain*
HYDRASTIS	*Viscous yellow discharge with pruritus*
KALIUM BICHROMICUM	*Ulcerative tendency*
MEDORRHINUM	*Previous urogenital infections; often chronic disorders*
MERCURIUS CORROSIVUS	*Ulceration with corrosive and blood-streaked leukorrhea*
MERCURIUS SOLUBILIS	*Profuse, greenish-yellow, irritant leukorrhea*
PULSATILLA	*Sometimes irritant leukorrhea*
SEPIA	*Sensation of pelvic heaviness "bearing-down"*
SILICEA	*Recurring and lingering infections*
SULFUR (SULPHUR)	*Burning irritation with fetid discharge*
THUYA (THUJA OCCIDENTALIS)	*Chronic disorders*

MUCUS-LIKE (Consistency)

BRONCHIAL

AMMONIUM CARBONICUM	*Bronchial obstruction with difficult expectoration during cardiorespiratory episodes*
ANTIMONIUM TARTARICUM	*Dyspnea with fluttering of nostrils, coated tongue*
ARSENICUM ALBUM	*Asthma or bronchitis with intense dyspnea, anxiety, aggravation between 1 and 3 a.m.*

COCCUS CACTI	
GRINDELIA	*Severe dyspnea with aggravation when going to bed or falling asleep*
KALIUM BICHROMICUM	
KALIUM CARBONICUM	*Asthma*
KALIUM IODATUM	*Severe respiratory disorders aggravated around 3 a.m. with irritating ENT discharge*
KALIUM MURIATICUM	*Viscous, difficult expectoration, with ENT signs*
LYCOPODIUM	*Fluttering of the nostrils during acute episodes, salty-tasting expectoration*
NATRUM MURIATICUM	
SENEGA	*Cough with dyspnea keeps patient from lying down; cough ending by sneezing*
SEPIA	

CONJUNCTIVA

ARGENTUM NITRICUM	*Intense pain*
EUPHRASIA	*Irritant eye-watering*
GRAPHITES	*Photophobia*
KALIUM BICHROMICUM	*Ulcerative tendency with filamentous secretions*
PULSATILLA	*Aggravation due to wind, abundant non-irritant eye-watering*
SEPIA	*Aggravation at night and due to fresh air*

DIGESTIVE

ACONITUM	
ALOE	*Gelatinous mucus with tenesmus and sphincter insecurity*
ARGENTUM NITRICUM	
ARSENICUM ALBUM	*Heartburn, craving for cold drinks that are rapidly vomited, alteration of general condition*
IPECA (IPECAC)	*Nausea and hypersalivation*
IRIS VERSICOLOR	*Heartburn and esophageal burning; frequent headaches*
KALIUM BICHROMICUM	*Filamentous mucus*
MERCURIUS SOLUBILIS	*Extensive tenesmus with sometimes bloody mucus*

ENT

ALUMINA	*Dryness of the mucous membranes with crusting when infected*
COCCUS CACTI	*Spasmodic nocturnal cough or aggravated when coming in from the cold, with posterior flow*
CORALLIUM RUBRUM	*Whooping-like cough with redness or cyanosis of the face during spasmodic coughing spells*
HYDRASTIS	
IPECA (IPECAC)	*Abundant salivation with nausea and sometimes vomiting, clean tongue*
KALIUM BICHROMICUM	*Thread-like discharge, sometimes bloody, posterior phlegm*

KALIUM MURIATICUM	*Milky-white mucus, viscous-like thick drool; context of eustachian tube catarrh; white or grayish coating of the posterior part of the tongue*
KALIUM SULFURICUM	*Transparent nasal mucus, thread-like, sometimes dark yellow or greenish-yellow; nasal blockage aggravated by heat with anosmia and ageusia*
NATRUM MURIATICUM	*"Egg-white" ENT and genital discharge*

GENITAL

BORAX	*"Egg-white" leukorrhea, context of genital ulcers*
BOVISTA	*Heavy menstruation with pronounced PMS*
CALCAREA PHOSPHORICA	*"Egg-white" leukorrhea*
KALIUM BICHROMICUM	
MEDORRHINUM	
MERCURIUS SOLUBILIS	*Irritant leukorrhea with intense nocturnal pruritus*
NATRUM MURIATICUM	*"Egg-white" leukorrhea alternating with bouts of vaginal dryness*
PULSATILLA	
SEPIA	
SILICEA	
SULFUR (SULPHUR)	*Irritant, fetid, burning discharge*
THUYA (THUJA OCCIDENTALIS)	

NASAL

ALLIUM CEPA	*Irritant nasal discharge improved by fresh air*
ARALIA RACEMOSA	*Rhinitis with irritant watery discharge, dry cough and asthma aggravated in the early night, sensitivity to drafts*
ARSENICUM ALBUM	*Scant watery catarrh, but burning greatly, excoriating the upper lip, improved by heat*
ARSENICUM IODATUM	*Watery discharge, burning, highly irritant, cervical adenopathy; sero-mucous otitis*
ARUM TRIPHYLLUM	*Bright red inflammation of the ENT mucous membranes with excoriation of the nostrils and upper lip, voice timbre varies during conversation, irritant and abundant saliva*
AURUM METALLICUM	*Fetid discharge*
BROMUM	*Watery and excoriating coryza; improved at seaside or at sea, hoarse cough*
CHAMOMILLA	*Mucous coryza when teething*
COCCUS CACTI	*Spasmodic nocturnal cough or aggravated when coming in from the cold, with postnasal drip*
CORALLIUM RUBRUM	*Spasmodic whooping-like cough with redness or cyanosis of the face during coughing spells*
DULCAMARA	*Posterior catarrh with sensation of stuffy nose, after exposure to damp cold or fog*
EUPHRASIA	*Irritant ocular discharge, improved by heat*
FERRUM PHOSPHORICUM	*Pale red epistaxis; otitis associated with rhinopharyngitis*
GRAPHITES	

HEPAR SULFUR	*Fetid greenish discharge*
HYDRASTIS	*Thick viscous yellow discharge, sometimes bloody*
IODUM	*Clear, irritant catarrh*
IPECA (IPECAC)	*Nasal obstruction, abundant salivation with nausea and sometimes vomiting, clean tongue; tendency towards epistaxis*
KALIUM BICHROMICUM	*Viscous discharge, transparent or yellowish sometimes streaked with blood, non-irritant; pain at the base of the teeth of the upper maxillary*
KALIUM IODATUM	*Abundant and irritant watery discharge with swollen and red nose; discharge rapidly becomes purulent; sensation of pressure at the base of the nose and frontal sinus pain; aggravation due to cold; ocular affection with red, swollen and watery eyes*
KALIUM MURIATICUM	*Milky-white mucus, viscous-like thick drool; context of eustachian tube catarrh, white or grayish coating on the posterior part of the tongue*
KALIUM SULFURICUM	*Transparent nasal mucus, flowing, sometimes dark yellow or greenish-yellow; nasal blockage aggravated by heat with anosmia and ageusia*
MERCURIUS SOLUBILIS	*Irritant and watery discharge at the beginning of coryza, sometimes bloody then purulent*
MEZEREUM	*Malar pain with thick and bloody nasal discharge*
NATRUM MURIATICUM	*"Egg-white" catarrh and abundant eye-watering alternating with dryness of the mucous membranes*
NUX VOMICA	*Clear and non-irritant catarrh during the day with plugged-up nose at night, and by heat; hypersensitivity to odors and drafts*
PHOSPHORUS	*Tendency towards epistaxis; alternation of dryness and watery catarrh; olfactory hypersensitivity*
PULSATILLA	*Recurring rhinopharyngitis and otitis in sensitive-type patients*
RUMEX CRISPUS	*Sensitivity to inhaling cold air*
SABADILLA	*Pruritus of the nose and soft palate; need to scratch ones nose*

SULFUR (SULPHUR)
SULFUR IODATUM (SULPHUR IODATUM)
SILICEA
SEPIA
THUYA (THUJA OCCIDENTALIS)

NON-IRRITANT

COCCUS CACTI
CORALLIUM RUBRUM
HYDRASTIS
KALIUM BICHROMICUM
KALIUM MURIATICUM
KALIUM SULFURICUM
NATRUM MURIATICUM

NUX VOMICA
PULSATILLA
SEPIA
THUYA (THUJA OCCIDENTALIS)

NOT ABUNDANT

See **ABSENCE (dryness of the mucous membranes)**

OCULAR

See **CONJUNCTIVA**

ORANGE

NATRUM CARBONICUM	*Rhinitis or diarrhea resembling orange pulp, in hot weather, aggravated by milk*

PHARYNGEAL

AILANTHUS	*Purple pharyngeal redness with ulceration; altered general condition, fetid discharge and breath, very sensitive and extensive cervical adenopathy; medicines for severe sore throat*
ARSENICUM ALBUM	*Alteration of the general condition, dry and red tongue; intense thirst; aggravated by drinking cold beverages*
ARUM TRIPHYLLUM	*Bright red pharynx, raspberry-like tongue, abundant saliva, alteration of the general condition; lips peel, and patient bites them until they bleed*
HEPAR SULFUR	*Medicine for all acute suppuration conditions*
KALIUM BICHROMICUM	*Thick and adhesive false membranes; ulceration on the pillars of the soft palate or the uvula with clear-cut edges, with viscous greenish-yellow mucus*
KALIUM MURIATICUM	*False membranes and grayish discharge*
MERCURIUS CYANATUS	*False membranes or thick discharge on the tonsils, marked dysphagia*
MERCURIUS SOLUBILIS	*Dysphagia, characteristic tongue and breath, viscous sweating during fever*

PURULENT

See **MUCOPURULENT**

SINUS

ACONITUM	*At the onset of fever, after a chill due to dry cold*
AURUM METALLICUM	*Chronic sinusitis*
BELLADONNA	*Throbbing, pulsating pain in the face and behind the eyes, facial redness, and hyperesthesia*

CINNABARIS (MERCURIUS SULPHURATUS RUBER)	*Peri-orbital pain of the frontal and maxillary sinuses, posterior flow*
CORALLIUM RUBRUM	*Frontal and maxillary sinus pain, congested face, aggravation when leaning forward, head-first*
HEPAR SULFUR	*Acute suppuration*
HYDRASTIS	*Aggravation of nasal blockage in hot rooms, posterior flow of the frontal and maxillary sinuses*
KALIUM BICHROMICUM	*Postnasal drip with painful upper maxillary, pain is felt at the base of the upper teeth*
KALIUM IODATUM	*Irritant nasal and ocular discharge, left sub-orbital headaches*
MERCURIUS SOLUBILIS	*Mucopurulent discharge irritating the nasal cavity*
MEZEREUM	*Bloody mucus, pain in the malar bones*
SILICEA	*Purulent discharge with maxillary pain*

STICKY

ELAPS	*Purulent discharge with fetid greenish crusts; mainly indicated in chronic otitis*
HYDRASTIS	*Burning pain along with yellowish discharge, mainly around nasal part of pharynx*
KALIUM BICHROMICUM	*Sticky thick discharge, gelatinous, greenish-yellow*
LYCOPODIUM	
MEZEREUM	*Acute coryza with pain in the malar area (nose and face bones), acute or chronic maxillary sinusitis*
THUYA (THUJA OCCIDENTALIS)	*Thick greenish-yellow discharge of all mucous membranes*

TRACHEAL

See **LARYNGEAL**

ULCERATIVE (With ulceration)

See **EXCORIATING**

VISCOUS

See also **STICKY**

ANTIMONIUM TARTARICUM	*Difficult expectoration, sometimes fluttering of the nostrils; paleness, cold sweating with cyanosis and sleepiness sometimes*
COCCUS CACTI	*Sometimes dry cough aggravated by heat and before midnight*
CORALLIUM RUBRUM	*Clear posterior catarrh*
ELAPS	*Purulent catarrh with fetid greenish crusts*

GRINDELIA	*Abundant discharge with difficult expectoration leading to choking*
HYDRASTIS	*Greenish-yellow*
KALIUM BICHROMICUM	*Greenish-yellow*
MEPHITIS PUTORIUS	*Whooping-like cough with laryngeal spasm*
PHELLANDRIUM	*Chronic pulmonary suppuration with abundant and fetid expectoration*
THUYA (THUJA OCCIDENTALIS)	*Chronic purulent discharge, thick, greenish of all mucous membranes*

WATERY (Like water)

CONJUNCTIVA

ALLIUM CEPA	*Non-irritant discharge*
ARGENTUM NITRICUM	*Splinter-like pain, photophobia and tendency to ulceration*
ARSENICUM ALBUM	*Burning sensation improved by heat*
BELLADONNA	*Conjunctive redness with photophobia*
EUPHRASIA	*Abundant and irritant eye-watering with photophobia*
KALIUM IODATUM	*Irritant eye-watering and nasal discharge, ulcerative conjunctivitis, aggravation due to fresh air and wind*
MERCURIUS SOLUBILIS	*Discharge rapidly becoming mucopurulent*
NAPHTALINUM	*Abundant and excoriating coryza, improved by fresh air, with irritant eye-watering*
SULFUR (SULPHUR)	

DIGESTIVE

ARSENICUM ALBUM	*Thirsty for small quantities of cold water, vomited once warmed in the stomach*
IRIS VERSICOLOR	*Gastroesophageal acid reflux with burns irradiating towards the throat and tip of the tongue, sometimes vomiting of thread-like mucus*
KREOSOTUM	*Gastritis with bloody vomiting*
MEZEREUM	*Inflammation of the tongue and entire digestive tube*
PHOSPHORUS	*Bloody vomiting, epigastric pain improved by drinking iced water. Painless diarrhea with discolored stools. Sensation that stools contain grains of rice*
RHEUM OFFICINALE	*Peri-umbilical pain when teething*
ROBINIA	*Gastroesophageal acid reflux with burns and acid vomiting*

GENITAL

BORAX	*Vaginal or genital ulceration, irritant leukorrhea*
FRAXINUS AMERICANA	*Abundant watery discharge with uterine fibroids and sensation of ptosis*

NASAL

ALLIUM CEPA	*Irritant nasal discharge improved by fresh air*
ARALIA RACEMOSA	*Rhinitis with watery, irritant discharge, dry cough and asthma, aggravated early in the evening, sensitivity to drafts*
ARSENICUM ALBUM	*Watery catarrh, scant but burning, excoriating the upper lip, improved by heat*
ARSENICUM IODATUM	*Watery discharge, burning, very irritant*
ARUM TRIPHYLLUM	*Bright red inflammation of the ENT mucous membranes with excoriation of the nostrils and upper lip, voice timbre varies during conversation; profuse and irritant salivation*
BELLADONNA	*Dry mucous membranes at the onset of acute episodes*
BROMUM	*Improved at seaside or at sea, hoarse cough*
CHAMOMILLA	
DULCAMARA	*Disorders occur if a chill is caught, or damp cold*
EUPHRASIA	*Irritant eye discharge, improved by heat*
IODUM	*Irritant discharge; laryngeal polarity; close to KALIUM IODATUM*
KALIUM IODATUM	*Watery discharge, irritant with swollen red nose, abundant then purulent; sensation of pressure at the base of the nose and sinus pain; aggravation due to cold; ocular disorder with red, puffy, watery eyes*
MERCURIUS SOLUBILIS	*Irritant and watery discharge at the beginning of coryza, sometimes bloody*
NAPHTALINUM	*Improved with fresh air*
NUX VOMICA	*After dryness of the mucous membranes at the onset of disorders; hypersensitivity to odors and drafts*
PHOSPHORUS	*Tendency to epistaxis; alternation of dryness and watery catarrh; olfactory hypersensitivity*
RUMEX CRISPUS	*Sensitivity to breathing in cold air*
SABADILLA	*Nose and soft palate pruritus, urge to rub ones nose*
SANGUINARIA CANADENSIS	*Nasal polyposis with anosmia and sometimes bloody discharge*
SANGUINARIA NITRICA	*Context of nasal polyposis with catarrh*

WHITE, Milky

ENT

KALIUM MURIATICUM	*White mucus like milk, viscous like thick drool, in a context of eustachian tube catarrh; white or grayish coating of the posterior part of the tongue*
MERCURIUS CYANATUS	*Severe throat inflammation with pultaceous coating and false membranes*

GENITAL

CALCAREA CARBONICA	*Leukorrhea*
GRAPHITES	*Irritant leukorrhea with pruritus*
HELONIAS DIOICA	*Leukorrhea resembling curdled milk*
PULSATILLA	*Thick yellowish leukorrhea, sometimes irritant*
SEPIA	*White or yellowish leukorrhea, excoriating and burning*
SILICEA	*Chronic leukorrhea*

2 - LACTATION

ABUNDANT

CALCAREA CARBONICA
LAC CANINUM

ENGORGED breast

APIS MELLIFICA	*Edema and burning improved by cold applications*
BELLADONNA	*Risk of abscess*
BORAX	*Thick milk that tastes bad*
BRYONIA	
CALCAREA CARBONICA	
LAC CANINUM	*Associated breast pain*
LACHESIS MUTUS	*Risk of abscess or lymphangitis*
PULSATILLA	
PYROGENIUM	*If infected*
RANA BUFO (BUFO RANA)	*Lymphangitis*
RICINUS	

GALACTORRHEA

PREGNANCY (During)

ASA FOETIDA

PREGNANCY (Outside of)

CHINA (CINCHONA)	
CONIUM	*Persistent galactorrhea after weaning*
CYCLAMEN	*Amenorrhea, galactorrhea*
MERCURIUS SOLUBILIS	
PHYTOLACCA	
PULSATILLA	*Occurring at the onset of puberty*
RICINUS	

INSUFFICIENT

ALFALFA	*Low dilutions*
CALCAREA CARBONICA	
CHINA	
RICINUS	*In medium dilutions, increases lactation during breastfeeding*

LYMPHANGITIS

APIS	*Pinkish-red edema*
BELLADONNA	*Throbbing pain with risk of abscess*
BRYONIA	*Pain aggravated by the slightest movement; great thirst*
LACHESIS MUTUS	*Risk of suppuration; livedo*

PHYTOLACCA	
PYROGENIUM	
RANA BUFO (BUFO RANA)	*Burning pain with painful lymph trajectory*
VIPERA REDI	*Painful indurated ropy veins*

WEANING (Help with)

LAC CANINUM	
PHYTOLACCA	*Pain at nipple level irradiating through the entire back, often with axillary adenopathy*
PULSATILLA	
RICINUS	*In this case use a high dilution*

3 - SALIVATION

ABUNDANT

AURUM METALLICUM	
CHAMOMILLA	
IGNATIA	
IPECA (IPECAC)	*Nausea with clean tongue and hypersalivation*
IRIS VERSICOLOR	
JABORANDI	*Hypersalivation with sensation of heat in the mouth*
KALIUM BICHROMICUM	
KREOSOTUM	
MERCURIUS SOLUBILIS	*Stomatitis, gingivitis or sore throat with characteristic tongue and breath*
NATRUM MURIATICUM	*Foamy saliva with bubbles lining the edge of the tongue*
NITRICUM ACIDUM	
PODOPHYLLUM	*Hyper-salivation when teething*
SULFURICUM ACIDUM (SULPHURICUM ACIDUM)	

Not very ABUNDANT with dry mouth

ACONITUM	
APIS	
ATROPINUM	
BELLADONNA	
BRYONIA	*Intense thirst for large quantities*
GELSEMIUM	
JABORANDI	*Administer in low dilutions, mother tincture*
NUX MOSCHATA	
PULSATILLA	

TASTE

ACID

ARGENTUM NITRICUM
CALCAREA CARBONICA
LYCOPODIUM
MAGNESIA CARBONICA
NUX VOMICA
PHOSPHORUS

BITTER

ACONITUM	*All food and drink, except water*
BRYONIA	*All food and drink, except water*
CHELIDONIUM	
CHINA	*All food and drink, event water*
NATRUM CARBONICUM	
NATRUM SULFURICUM	
NUX VOMICA	

PULSATILLA
SULFUR (SULPHUR)

METALLIC

COCCULUS	*Motion sickness, nausea during pregnancy*
MERCURIUS SOLUBILIS	*Abundant salivation, viscous, with thirst*

SALTY

CARBO VEGETABILIS	
CYCLAMEN	
LYCOPODIUM	
NATRUM MURIATICUM	*Abundant and salty salivation alternating with a sensation of dry mouth*
PHOSPHORUS	
SEPIA	
SULFUR (SULPHUR)	

4 - SWEATING

ABUNDANT

ANTIMONIUM TARTARICUM	
ARSENICUM ALBUM	*Sweating when falling asleep, algid; and cold sweating in acute conditions*
BELLADONNA	*Sweating in acute feverish conditions with redness of the face*
BRYONIA	*Progressive onset of fever*
CALCAREA CARBONICA	
CARBO VEGETABILIS	
CHINA (CINCHONA)	*Intense thirst and asthenia*
FERRUM METALLICUM	*Fever*
HEPAR SULFUR	*Sweating at the slightest effort*
JABORANDI	*Hypersalivation*
KALIUM CARBONICUM	*Sweating at the slightest effort, cardiorespiratory disorders*
MERCURIUS SOLUBILIS	*Sweating aggravated at night during acute conditions, viscous sweating*
NATRUM MURIATICUM	*Fever and headache improved by sweating*
OPIUM	*Profuse sweating whereas any discharge is diminished*
PHOSPHORICUM ACIDUM	*Nocturnal sweating mainly in asthenic patients*
PSORINUM	*Profuse fetid sweating following an acute condition*
SAMBUCCUS	*Abundant facial sweating when waking; disappears when falling back to sleep*
SEPIA	
SILICEA	*Fetid and cold sweating mostly on the extremities*
SULFUR (SULPHUR)	
THUYA (THUJA OCCIDENTALIS)	*Viscous sweat, strong odor, aggravation when falling asleep*
TUBERCULINUM	*Sweating at the slightest effort and during fever, even slight fever, and sleep*
VERATRUM ALBUM	*Lipothymia with cold sweating during toxic-infectious syndromes or certain dysmenorrhea episodes*
VERATRUM VIRIDE	*Hot, viscous sweating in plethoric, congestive patients*

AGGRAVATION of the general condition (With)

ARSENICUM ALBUM	
CHAMOMILLA	
CHINA (CINCHONA)	*Tiring sweating that provides no relief*
HEPAR SULFUR	*Profuse in acute conditions with coughing*
MERCURIUS SOLUBILIS	
OPIUM	
PHOSPHORUS	
RHUS TOXICODENDRON	

ALTERNATION of sweating and skin dryness

APIS	*With fever*
KALIUM CARBONICUM	

ARMPITS

IODUM	
KALIUM CARBONICUM	
NITRICUM ACIDUM	*Fetid and excoriating sweating*
PETROLEUM	
SEPIA	*Fetid and excoriating sweating*
SULFUR (SULPHUR)	*Strong-smelling and irritant sweat*
THUYA (THUJA OCCIDENTALIS)	*Strong-smelling sweat, smelling of leeks*

COLD

ANTIMONIUM TARTARICUM	*With a vaso-vagal syndrome*
ARSENICUM ALBUM	
BARYTA CARBONICA	*Cold sweating of the feet*
CALCAREA CARBONICA	*Sweating with a sensation of cold*
CALCAREA PHOSPHORICA	
CARBO VEGETABILIS	*Found in respiratory disorders with cyanosis and a pre-collapse state, sweating is mostly on the face and forehead*
CHINA (CINCHONA)	
COCCULUS	
IPECA (IPECAC)	*With a vaso-vagal syndrome*
LOBELIA INFLATA	*With nausea and fainting; asthma*
NAJA NAJA (NAJA TRIPUDIANS)	*With cyanosis of the extremities, and hot face*
RHEUM OFFICINALE	*Localized on the face*
SILICEA	*With acute and chronic conditions*
STRAMONIUM	*During convulsions*
TABACUM	*Motion sickness, facial sweating with associated vaso-vagal syndrome*
TUBERCULINUM	*Headaches with vomiting*
VERATRUM ALBUM	*During acute infectious episodes, in a fainting context, localized on the forehead*

CONVALESCENCE (During)

CHINA (CINCHONA)	*Nocturnal aggravation*
PSORINUM	*Profuse sweating following acute diseases*

COUGH (During)

HEPAR SULFUR	*Profuse sweating without relief*

EFFORT (At the slightest)

CALCAREA CARBONICA	*Mostly around the head*

CHINA (CINCHONA)	
GRAPHITES	
HEPAR SULFUR	*Essentially during feverish conditions, following a cough*
IODUM	
KALIUM CARBONICUM	*Abundant sweating with cardiorespiratory disorders; sometimes lack of sweat*
PHOSPHORUS	*During acute conditions*
SEPIA	
SULFUR (SULPHUR)	
TUBERCULINUM	

EMOTIONS (Due to)

AMBRA GRISEA	*Sweating when talking*
ARGENTUM NITRICUM	
BARYTA CARBONICA	*In front of strangers*
GELSEMIUM	*Anxiety and following a fright*
IGNATIA	
OPIUM	*Mostly following a fright*
PULSATILLA	*With flushed face*
PSORINUM	
SEPIA	*Localized in the armpits; aggravated when writing*
SILICEA	*Cold sweating on the extremities*
SULFUR (SULPHUR)	

FEET

BARYTA CARBONICA	
CALCAREA CARBONICA	*Cold feet*
FLUORICUM ACIDUM	
GRAPHITES	*Intermittent and fetid*
IODUM	
KALIUM CARBONICUM	
LYCOPODIUM	*Cold and profuse*
NITRICUM ACIDUM	
PETROLEUM	*Fetid*
PSORINUM	*Viscous sweating*
SEPIA	*Irritating the toes, and fetid*
SILICEA	*Fetid and irritant mostly in between toes*
SULFUR (SULPHUR)	

FETID

BARYTA CARBONICA	*Sweating of the feet; sweat is cold*
GRAPHITES	*On feet, only when there is general skin dryness*
HEPAR SULFUR	*Acrid and foul-smelling odor*
KALIUM CARBONICUM	*Fetid sweating of the feet*
NITRICUM ACIDUM	*Armpits and feet*
PSORINUM	*Viscous and fetid*
SEPIA	
SILICEA	*Irritant, foul-smelling, fetid and cold sweating of the feet*

SULFUR (SULPHUR) — *Smelling of rot*
THUYA (THUJA OCCIDENTALIS) — *Foul-smelling, oily and greasy sweating*

FRIGHT (Following a)

See **EMOTIONS**

GENERALIZED

ARSENICUM ALBUM	
HEPAR SULFUR	*At the slightest effort and in acute feverish conditions*
KALIUM CARBONICUM	*At the slightest effort*
MERCURIUS SOLUBILIS	*Skin is always clammy*
NITRICUM ACIDUM	
SEPIA	*Hyper-hidrosis of the hands and armpits*
SILICEA	*Generally localized sweating, sometimes generalized during suppurations*
SULFUR (SULPHUR)	

GENITAL

GELSEMIUM	*Scrotum*
LYCOPODIUM	
MERCURIUS SOLUBILIS	
PETROLEUM	
SEPIA	*Constant*
SULFUR (SULPHUR)	
THUYA (THUJA OCCIDENTALIS)	*Fetid and faintly-smelling sweating*

GOING TO SLEEP (When)

ARSENICUM ALBUM	*In acute conditions*
CALCAREA PHOSPHORICA	*Associated to weakness*
CONIUM MACULATUM	*On falling asleep and continuing throughout sleep*
SILICEA	
THUYA (THUJA OCCIDENTALIS)	*At the beginning of sleep*

HANDS

CALCAREA CARBONICA	
IGNATIA	*Due to emotion*
IODUM	
PSORINUM	*Palms of the hands*
SEPIA	*When writing, dyshidrosis*
SILICEA	*While writing*
SULFUR (SULPHUR)	

HEAD

IN GENERAL

CALCAREA CARBONICA *At the slightest effort, mostly the scalp*
CALCAREA PHOSPHORICA *Mostly nocturnal sweating*

EYEBROWS

THUYA (THUJA OCCIDENTALIS)

FACE

CALCAREA CARBONICA
CALCAREA PHOSPHORICA
KALIUM CARBONICUM
MERCURIUS SOLUBILIS
SILICEA

FOREHEAD

CALCAREA CARBONICA
VERATRUM ALBUM *Sweating of the forehead during acute conditions*

NAPE OF THE NECK

SILICEA
SULFUR (SULPHUR)

NECK

CALCAREA PHOSPHORICA
SILICEA *And of the scalp*
SULFUR (SULPHUR)

NOSE

NATRUM MURIATICUM
THUYA (THUJA OCCIDENTALIS)
Localized on the nostrils

OCCIPUT

CALCAREA CARBONICA *Abundant cold sweating*
SILICEA

UPPER LIP

SEPIA
THUYA (THUJA OCCIDENTALIS)

HOT

BELLADONNA *With fever*
BRYONIA *With fever*

CHAMOMILLA	*Around the head and face*
OPIUM	*Sweating observed during acute intoxication*
PHOSPHORUS	*Sweating and hyperthermia in acute pulmonary conditions*
VERATRUM VIRIDE	*Hot and profuse sweating*

IMPROVEMENT of the general condition by sweating

ACONITUM	
BRYONIA	
GELSEMIUM	*With fever*
LYCOPODIUM	*With fever*
NATRUM MURIATICUM	*Feverish syndrome and headache improved by sweating*
PSORINUM	*Can sweat profusely following acute diseases; if so, sweating improves the general condition*
SULFUR (SULPHUR)	*Acid and foul-smelling sweating*

IRRITANT

BARYTA CARBONICA	*Feet*
FLUORICUM ACIDUM	*Excoriating, mostly in between toes*
NITRICUM ACIDUM	
SEPIA	*Irritant and foul-smelling*
SILICEA	*Fetid, mostly around the feet*
SULFUR (SULPHUR)	

MISSING

ACONITUM	*No sweating during fever*
ALUMINA	*General dryness of the skin and mucous membranes*
GRAPHITES	*No sweating on the body; the skin is dry, but fetid sweating of the feet*
KALIUM CARBONICUM	*May have an incapacity to sweat*
LYCOPODIUM	*With age, sweating can subside*
NUX VOMICA	
PETROLEUM	*Skin dryness in general but localized sweating*
PSORINUM	*The skin is normally dry, but there can be localized sweating*

NIGHTTIME

BARYTA CARBONICA	
CALCAREA PHOSPHORICA	*Of the head*
HEPAR SULFUR	
KALIUM CARBONICUM	*Mostly after midnight*
MERCURIUS SOLUBILIS	
PHOSPHORICUM ACIDUM	
PHOSPHORUS	
PULSATILLA	
SEPIA	
SILICEA	

THUYA (THUJA OCCIDENTALIS)
TUBERCULINUM

ODOR

ACID, Sour-smelling

HEPAR SULFUR
NATRUM PHOSPHORICUM
SULFUR (SULPHUR)
SULFURICUM ACIDUM (SULPHURICUM ACIDUM)

ACRID

BRYONIA
CALCAREA CARBONICA
HEPAR SULFUR
MAGNESIA CARBONICA
NATRUM PHOSPHORICUM
RHEUM OFFICINALE

BLAND

THUYA (THUJA OCCIDENTALIS)

FETID

GRAPHITES
KALIUM PHOSPHORICUM
PETROLEUM *Mostly armpits and feet*
PSORINUM
SEPIA
SILICEA
SULFUR (SULPHUR)

FOUL-SMELLING

BARYTA CARBONICA *Feet*
FLUORICUM ACIDUM
GRAPHITES
HEPAR SULFUR
LYCOPODIUM
MERCURIUS SOLUBILIS
NITRICUM ACIDUM
SEPIA
SILICEA
SULFUR (SULPHUR)

GARLIC, Smelling of leeks

BOVISTA
THUYA (THUJA OCCIDENTALIS)

SWEET and SOUR

THUYA (THUJA OCCIDENTALIS)

OILY

BRYONIA
MERCURIUS SOLUBILIS
NATRUM MURIATICUM
PSORINUM
SELENIUM

PARTIAL

CALCAREA CARBONICA	*Cold and localized*
KALIUM CARBONICUM	*On the painful area*
PSORINUM	*Palms of the hands*
PULSATILLA	*Localized and unilateral*

PERINEUM

LYCOPODIUM
MERCURIUS SOLUBILIS
PETROLEUM
SEPIA
SULFUR (SULPHUR)
THUYA (THUJA OCCIDENTALIS)

SLEEP (During)

CALCAREA CARBONICA	*Wets the pillow*
CHINA (CINCHONA)	*Abundant and tiring*
CONIUM MACULATUM	
SILICEA	
THUYA (THUJA OCCIDENTALIS)	
TUBERCULINUM	

STAINING clothes with yellow

MERCURIUS SOLUBILIS
NITRICUM ACIDUM
TUBERCULINUM

TIRING

CALCAREA PHOSPHORICA
CHINA (CINCHONA)
PSORINUM

UNCOVERED AREAS (Around)

PULSATILLA	*Mostly unilateral and fetid, cold*
THUYA (THUJA OCCIDENTALIS)	*In acute conditions*

UPPER PART OF THE BODY (Never the lower part)

CALCAREA CARBONICA *Mostly head and neck*

VISCOUS

MERCURIUS SOLUBILIS
PSORINUM

WAKING UP (When)

SAMBUCUS *Profuse sweating on awakening that stops when falling asleep again; dry skin during the night*

SULFUR (SULPHUR)
THUYA (THUJA OCCIDENTALIS) *Sweating during sleep; improved when waking up*

WRITING (While)

SEPIA
SILICEA

5 - MENSTRUATION

ABSENCE OF PERIODS: *Amenorrhea*

ACONITUM	*Often following a fright*
AURUM METALLICUM	*Secondary amenorrhea with depression*
CALCAREA CARBONICA	*Delayed puberty*
FERRUM METALLICUM	*General anemic tendency*
GRAPHITES	*Delayed puberty or pre-menopause hormonal deficiency*
IGNATIA	*Following an emotional shock*
KALIUM CARBONICUM	*Primary or secondary amenorrhea*
LACHESIS MUTUS	*Pre-menopause amenorrhea with characteristic circulatory disorders*
LYCOPODIUM	*Amenorrhea due to oral contraception*
MOSCHUS	*Following a fright*
NATRUM MURIATICUM	*Secondary pubertal amenorrhea sometimes following an emotional shock*
PHOSPHORUS	*Amenorrhea with epistaxis*
PULSATILLA	*Associated peripheral venous circulatory disorders*
SENECIO AUREUS	*Absence of menstruation, with vicariate disorders*
SEPIA	*Sensation of pelvic heaviness, hot flashes with sweating*

ABUNDANT: *Menorrhagia*

ACTAEA RACEMOSA (CIMICIFUGA)	*With spasmodic pain proportional to blood flow, agitation and fainting tendency*
ARNICA	*Menorrhagia by first-generation IUD*
AURUM MURIATICUM KALINATUM (AURUM MURIATICUM NATRONATUM)	*Uterine fibroid with menorrhagia*
BOVISTA	*With inter-menstrual syndrome (painful ovulation) and PMS; sensation of bloating in the abdomen; edema of the fingers*
CALCAREA CARBONICA	
CALCAREA PHOSPHORICA	*Painful and abundant blood flow*
CHAMOMILLA	*With unbearable pain*
CHINA (CINCHONA)	*Tiring dark blood meno-/metrorrhagia with clotting*
COCCULUS	*Painful periods with fainting, nausea and dizziness*
COCCUS CACTI	*Coagulated filamentous black blood with intense pain*
CROCUS SATIVUS	*Coagulated filamentous black blood*
CYCLAMEN	*Mostly abundant blood flow; previous to the onset of menstruation: ophthalmic headaches and dizziness*
ERIGERON	*Red blood; aggravated by movement*
FERRUM METALLICUM	*Clear and flowing blood; mainly iron deficiency anemia*
IPECA (IPECAC)	*Bright red blood with nausea and lipothymia*
KALIUM CARBONICUM	*Meno-/metrorrhagia followed by constant spotting*
MILLEFOLIUM	*General tendency to bleed heavily*
MUREX	*Painful heavy-bleeding periods, pain around the pubic symphysis*

PHOSPHORUS	*General tendency to bleed heavily*
SABINA	*Bright red blood with clots, sacrolumbar pain*
SECALE CORNUTUM	*Red blood with dark clotting, cramp pain*
TRILLIUM PENDULUM	*Heavy periods, with short cycles, pelvic pain, aggravation of blood flow and pain by movement, fainting syndrome*
TUBERCULINUM	*Abundant and long-lasting periods, painful, with short cycles*
VERATRUM ALBUM	*Heavy periods with fainting, cold sweating, diarrhea*

CLOSE together, early: *Short cycles*

AMBRA GRISEA	*Periods return at the slightest emotion*
AURUM MURIATICUM KALINATUM (AURUM MURIATICUM NATRONATUM)	*Context of uterine fibroid with menorrhagia*
CALCAREA CARBONICA	*Periods return at the slightest emotion*
CALCAREA PHOSPHORICA	*Or on the contrary: lengthy cycles*
ERIGERON	*Tendency to heavy bleeding, bright red blood aggravated by movement*
FERRUM METALLICUM	*Pale, abundant, intermittent, tiring blood flow, with headaches and hot flashes*
IPECA (IPECAC)	*Bright red blood flow with nausea and vomiting*
LILIUM TIGRINUM	*Sometimes amenorrhea; characteristic behavior; palpitations and hypotension*
MILLEFOLIUM	*Early, red-blood periods, abundant and lengthy*
PHOSPHORUS	
SABINA	*Red blood with dark clotting, paroxysmal lumbar and uterine pain*
SILICEA	*Abundant blood flow, notions of asthenia and cold-sensitivity*
THLASPI BURSA PASTORIS	*Early periods, abundant and lengthy, dark blood with large clots*
TRILLIUM PENDULUM	*Periods every 2 weeks, abundant and lengthy, lasting 6 days or more*
TUBERCULINUM	*Painful, abundant and lengthy periods*

CLOTS Abundant

ARGENTUM NITRICUM	*Right ovarian pain*
BELLADONNA	*Dark clots*
BOVISTA	*Flow of dark coagulated blood mostly at night, with diarrhea before and during menstruation*
CACTUS	*Constrictive pain in the uterus*
CALCAREA CARBONICA	
CALCAREA PHOSPHORICA	
CHAMOMILLA	*Abundant dark red blood flow, painful*
CHINA (CINCHONA)	*Anemic tendency, fainting with a need for fresh air*
COCCUS CACTI	*Filamentous blood flow*
CROCUS SATIVUS	*Dark clots with an aspect of "tarred strings"*
CYCLAMEN	

HAMAMELIS	
LACHESIS MUTUS	*Improvement of the general condition by black blood flow that looks like "chopped burnt straw"*
PLATINA	
PULSATILLA	
SABINA	*Dark blood with dark clots, paroxysmal lumbar and uterine pain*
SECALE	*Cramps and paresthesia*

DARK

CHINA (CINCHONA)	
CROCUS SATIVUS	*Abundant blood flow, partially coagulated blood with clots, aggravated by movement*
HAMAMELIS	*Black blood without clotting with ovarian and lumbar pain and pelvic numbness*
LACHESIS MUTUS	*Classically black blood flow with a"chopped burnt straw" aspect*
SECALE CORNUTUM	*Spasmodic uterine pain*
SEPIA	*Pelvic congestion with sensation of heaviness*
THLASPI BURSA PASTORIS	*Dark blood flow with large clots, abundant, lengthy and painful periods*
USTILAGO	*Black blood with clotting and filamentous aspect, intermittent spotting, gynecological bleeding at the slightest touch*

INSUFFICIENT: *Little blood flow*

CAULOPHYLLUM	*Intermittent pain with scant blood flow*
CONIUM	*Uterine fibroids*
GRAPHITES	*Widely-spaced periods, light-colored blood*
LACHESIS MUTUS	*With general aggravation*
PULSATILLA	*Insufficient, widely-spaced periods, intermittent dark red blood flow; late-onset puberty*
SENECIO AUREUS	*Insufficient or no periods*

PAINFUL

ACTAEA RACEMOSA (CIMICIFUGA)	*Spasmodic pain proportional to blood flow with agitation and fainting tendency*
BELLADONNA	
BORAX	*General hyperesthesia*
BOVISTA	*Black coagulated blood flow mostly at night, with diarrhea before and during menstruation*
BRYONIA	*Uterine pain with stinging right ovarian pain, improved by strong pressure and complete rest*
CACTUS	
CALCAREA PHOSPHORICA	
CAULOPHYLLUM	*Intermittent pain, with scant blood flow*
CHAMOMILLA	*Intense pain with agitation, clots that are difficult to expulse*

COCCULUS	*Spasms, dark blood flow, fainting tendency*
COLOCYNTHIS	*Spasmodic pain improved when doubled over and by strong pressure*
CUPRUM METALLICUM	*With copper IUD*
FOLLICULINUM	
IGNATIA	
KALIUM CARBONICUM	
LAC CANINUM	*Ovarian pain before periods, changing sides, with premenstrual mastodynia*
LACHESIS MUTUS	*Before cycles become regular*
LILIUM TIGRINUM	*Extreme pelvic heaviness, need to press the vulva with hands, throbbing ovarian pain irradiating towards the thighs*
LUTEINUM	*Membranous dysmenorrhea*
MAGNESIA CARBONICA	*Mostly nocturnal flow*
MAGNESIA PHOSPHORICA	*Uterine pain radiating towards the back, aggravated at night, improved by strong pressure; onset of pain one or two days before periods*
MUREX	*Heavy periods with big clots, pubic symphysis pain, pelvic heaviness improved when sitting with legs crossed*
NUX VOMICA	*With irritability, improved by heat*
PLATINA	*Dysmenorrhea with general and genital hyperesthesia*
PULSATILLA	*Late periods, not very abundant, intermittent, more abundant in daytime than at night*
SECALE CORNUTUM	*At the slightest movement with lengthy and abundant periods with non-coagulated black blood*
SEPIA	*Pelvic heaviness, numbness of the lumbar area, improved by sitting with legs crossed*
STAPHYSAGRIA	*Pain and fatigue in the lower limbs, hypersensitivity of the vulva to contact with fabric.*
TRILLIUM PENDULUM	*Sensation of dislocation of the pelvis and pubic and sacroiliac symphysis, improved by contention or a strong girdle.*
VERATRUM ALBUM	*Heavy periods with lipothymia, cold sweating, diarrhea*
VIBURNUM OPULUS	*Late periods and short-lived nausea, pollakiuria, uterine cramping with lipothymia, sacral pain radiating towards the pelvis and thighs*

RED: *Blood flow*

ARNICA	*Pelvic pain, flow not influenced by movement*
BELLADONNA	*With dark clotting*
CINNAMOMUM	*Bright red blood*
ERIGERON	*Bleeding in spurts, aggravated by movement*
FERRUM METALLICUM	*Context of anemia and asthenia on the general level with localized congestion*
IPECA (IPECAC)	
MILLEFOLIUM	*Tendency toward heavy bleeding, blood flow not aggravated by movement*

PHOSPHORUS	*Heavy and frequent periods*
SABINA	*Lumbar pain and at the front of thighs, dark clots*
TRILLIUM PENDULUM	*Aggravation due to movement, and considerable pelvic pain*

SPACED, LATE: *Lengthy cycles*

BARYTA CARBONICA	*Endocrine insufficiency*
CALCAREA CARBONICA	*Delayed-onset puberty*
CALCAREA PHOSPHORICA	*Or to the contrary: short cycles*
GRAPHITES	*Pale blood, endocrine insufficiency*
NATRUM MURIATICUM	*Sometimes secondary amenorrhea*
PULSATILLA	*In general late puberty, blood flow stops one day to start again the next; main blood flow during the day; variability of symptoms*
SENECIO AUREUS	*With cough in case of late periods*
VIBURNUM OPULUS	*Spasmodic dysmenorrhea with fainting, pain comes before menstruation*

CRAVINGS AND AVERSIONS

"*Tell me what you eat, and I'll tell you who you are*". In this well-known saying, Brillat-Savarin emphasizes the fact that our eating habits are an integral part of our cultural identity. Just as newborn babies seem marked by a spontaneous oral nature essential to development ("*All constructive affective exchanges are built around satisfying digestive experiences*" wrote Françoise Dolto), our eating habits are rapidly shaped by various factors:

- **Region and environment**: in cold and continental countries, foods are high in fats, and rich (stews, sauerkraut and starches); in warm southern European countries there is the famous Mediterranean diet with its vegetable oils, vegetables and fruit.

- **Family upbringing establishes** dietary requirements and abstentions via food choices, but also via culinary practices (we think of PULSATILLA patients who cook just like their mothers).

- **Social environment and friends**: while physicians are involved in dietary choices for children, when children become teenagers they wants to eat what their friends are eating, with a definite preference for food advertised on television. The cereals market has sky-rocketed and the consumption of ketchup has doubled in children under 5 since 1980 (Bensoussan: "*Ce que manger veut dire*"). Social backgrounds often lead to drastically varying eating choices.

- **Culture, race and religion**: for example, rice and strong spices are a given in Asian countries. Rituals and forbidden foods also shape eating habits: like pork in Muslim countries or alcohol in France which still has a rather male connotation. Finally what would a British person do if served frogs legs, or a European do if faced with a well-cooked dog or grilled insects!

Food is a strong cultural marker. Although our sense of taste is set at a very young age, it is still shaped by our environment. However, it is relatively difficult to change eating habits once adulthood is reached.

This long introduction was necessary to position and analyze this section on "**Food cravings and aversions**". These are classically listed with general symptoms. Often highly ranked, on the same level as characteristic mental symptoms, they are only of value when they are spontaneously expressed, showing an instinctive attitude, free from parasitic aspects of our food culture.
In some materia medica, cravings and aversions are listed under the heading "STOMACH".

Cravings have a greater value than aversions. In fact, according to Denis Demarque, three situations can be defined:

- Cravings can occur during acute affections. These are then concomitant symptoms, disappearing when patients improve. Thirst, a highly characteristic element, is reviewed in the "**Sensations**" chapter. It seemed excessive, however, to systematically list cravings and aversions among concomitant symptoms, as was the case in some materia medicas.

- Variations are due to physiopathological causes. They denote a chronic dysfunction that sometimes disappears after treatment. The ambivalence of NATRUM MURIATICUM, sometimes worsened by salt, is a good example.

- The eating preferences of a patient in equilibrium, with no real pathological disorders, correspond to the patient's physiology. They remain good indicators of a patient and of that patient's corresponding in-depth medicine, with certain reservations as stated above.

In any case, craving for salty, sweet, acidic as well as hot or cold foods remains a distinctly reliable element.

Aversions are less indicative. They most often are a manifestation of food intolerance, or even real allergy (eggs for FERRUM METALLICUM, fish for PHOSPHORUS). Thus, if PULSATILLA or CYCLAMEN subjects reject fatty foods, it is because they lead to dyspeptic disorders for one, and headaches for the other. It might be presumed that bread increases the flatulent colitis of CHINA subjects (CINCHONA), whereas in SILICEA subjects' aversion to breast milk, this is also due to intolerance.

Spontaneous aversion, without any link to a pathological disorder, remains relatively rare.

FOOD CRAVINGS

ACID

ANTIMONIUM CRUDUM	*Sour wine and vinegar. Mostly poorly tolerated with watery diarrhea and acid eructation*
HEPAR SULFUR	*Craving for vinegar sometimes*
PULSATILLA	*Craving for pickles, vinegar and sour fruit*
SEPIA	*Craving for mustard, pickles, vinegar and any sour food. This very common symptom is almost a keynote*
SULFUR (SULPHUR)	*Likes salad with plenty of dressing*
VERATRUM ALBUM	*Fruit and sour foods, aggravation of digestive disorders in acute cases*

ALCOHOL

AGARICUS MUSCARIUS	*Often leads to alcoholism*
AURUM METALLICUM	*Mostly in depressive conditions. Frequent alcoholism*
KALIUM BICHROMICUM	*Great craving for beer, not tolerated, digestive disorders*
LACHESIS MUTUS	*Mostly craving for wine. In men and women. Almost always found but not necessarily synonymous with alcoholism*
LUESINUM (SYPHILINUM)	
LYCOPODIUM	*Craves it but can't tolerate it well, especially mixing various alcohols. Often a "connaisseur"*
MEDORRHINUM	*Craving for alcohol at a young age, mostly teen years*
NUX VOMICA	*Strong craving for all stimulants, coffee, alcohol, tobacco, spicy food, pickles. Drinks much alcohol, dependent at first then secondly intolerant, with gastralgia and irritated colon*
SULFUR (SULPHUR)	*Enjoys drinking and likes fine spirits*
SULFURICUM ACIDUM (SULPHURICUM ACIDUM)	*Marked craving. Alcoholism with pyrosis and pancreatitis. Water is not tolerated*

BITTER drinks

NATRUM MURIATICUM
SEPIA

CHOCOLATE Dark

LYCOPODIUM	*Increases bloating*
SEPIA	*Very frequent craving in spite of not being attracted to sweets in general*
SULFUR (SULPHUR)	*Subject loves all types of sweets*

COFFEE

AURUM METALLICUM — *Aggravation of insomnia*
CHAMOMILLA — *Worsens nervous disorders*
NUX VOMICA

COLD

DRINKS

See also **THIRST** in the **SENSATIONS** chapter

ARSENICUM ALBUM — *Is sometimes found in acute conditions but is worsened*
CAUSTICUM — *Doesn't like water, cold drinks improve hoarseness and gastralgia*
PHOSPHORUS — *Craving for cold drinks in acute states. Vomited as soon as warmed up in the stomach*
PULSATILLA — *Craving for fizzy and sour drinks*
VERATRUM ALBUM

FOODS

PHOSPHORUS — *Imperious hunger after meals, at night*
PULSATILLA — *Craving for fresh, sour foods; juicy fruit*

CONDIMENTS

See **SPICY FOODS**

DAIRY PRODUCTS

CALCAREA CARBONICA — *All dairy products, in large quantities*
MERCURIUS SOLUBILIS
RHUS TOXICODENDRON — *Cold milk during an infection*
SILICEA — *Aggravation, mostly digestive*
TUBERCULINUM — *Cold milk*

EGGS

CALCAREA CARBONICA — *Strong craving, mostly in children*

FATTY (Foods)

ANTIMONIUM CRUDUM — *Pork and processed meats*
ARSENICUM ALBUM — *Rarely encountered*
CALCAREA PHOSPHORICA — *Smoked ham*
MERCURIUS SOLUBILIS — *Frequently craves butter*
NITRICUM ACIDUM — *Sausage, bacon, herring. Frequent symptoms. In general eats little meat*
NUX VOMICA — *Craving for fatty foods. Found sometimes in infectious states*
SULFUR (SULPHUR) — *Frequent, even eats the fat off someone else's plate!*
TUBERCULINUM — *Cold milk, smoked ham, bacon*

FRUIT

PHOSPHORICUM ACIDUM	*Aggravates diarrhea, painless most of the time*
PULSATILLA	
VERATRUM ALBUM	*Craving for sour fruit*

HOT (Drinks and food)

ARSENICUM ALBUM	*Finds comfort in hot drinks and foods for all disorders even burns. Likes hot and very hot food; reliable and frequent symptom*
CHELIDONIUM	*Improves digestive disorders*
LYCOPODIUM	*For adult and elderly patients*

ICE CREAM

ANTIMONIUM CRUDUM	*Diarrhea*
CALCAREA CARBONICA	
PHOSPHORUS	*Very pronounced*
PULSATILLA	*Poorly tolerated*

INDIGESTIBLE OR NON-EDIBLE FOODS

This particular behavior is mostly found in children. It can be dirt, plaster, clay, raw food (potatoes, rice). Of course children who put everything into their mouths by oral reflex do not count!

CALCAREA CARBONICA	*Frequent*
NITRICUM ACIDUM	
SILICEA	

OYSTERS

LYCOPODIUM	*Badly tolerated in general*
NATRUM MURIATICUM	*Frequent*

PICKLES Marinated

PULSATILLA	*Rare*
SEPIA	*Frequently encountered*
SULFUR (SULPHUR)	

SALT, Salty foods

ARGENTUM NITRICUM	*Not as common as craving for sweets*
CALCAREA PHOSPHORICA	*Frequent. Smoked and salty meat and fish*
CAUSTICUM	*Smoked foods*
NATRUM MURIATICUM	*Craving for smoked fish. The craving for salt is generally very strong, even in small children who lick the salt shakers; this is a keynote. Sometimes the children become disgusted by it, maybe by saturation*
NITRICUM ACIDUM	*Herring*
PHOSPHORUS	*Except fish and oysters*

SPICY FOODS

CAPSICUM	
NUX VOMICA	*Systematically seasons food: pepper, mustard, hot sauce. Frequent gastric disorders and colitis*
PULSATILLA	
SEPIA	*Likes all spices, like mustard, within reason. Good tolerance*
SULFUR (SULPHUR)	*Particularly likes very spicy and hot food. Frequent hemorrhoids*

STARCHES

CALCAREA CARBONICA	*Eats large quantities of potatoes, pasta and cereals. Craving more pronounced in children*

SWEETS

ARGENTUM NITRICUM	*Very frequent, aggravation of burning gastralgia*
CALCAREA CARBONICA	*Cakes*
CINA	*Ravenous hunger after meals or at night*
GRAPHITES	*Rare, aversion is more common*
KALIUM CARBONICUM	*Very pronounced*
LYCOPODIUM	*Need to snack on sweets*
SULFUR (SULPHUR)	*Eats too many sweets. Frequent hypoglycemia at the end of the morning*

FOOD AVERSIONS

ALCOHOL

CARBO VEGETABILIS	*By intolerance. Triggers congestive flashes and dyspeptic disorders*
LYCOPODIUM	*Caution and suspicion*

BREAD

CHINA (CINCHONA)	*Aggravation of bloating*
NATRUM MURIATICUM	*Rare*
NATRUM SULFURICUM	*Poor digestion of starches and carbohydrates*

EGGS

FERRUM METALLICUM	*Due to intolerance or allergy (?)*
SULFUR (SULPHUR)	*Sometimes*

FATTY (Foods)

CARBO VEGETABILIS	*Intolerance, with dyspepsia and bloating of the upper abdomen*
CYCLAMEN	*Mostly butter which induces headaches and migraines*
LYCOPODIUM	*Hepatic intolerance*
NATRUM MURIATICUM	
PULSATILLA	*Severe disgust and intolerance to butter, pork, processed meats leading to dyspeptic disorders*
SEPIA	*Frequent diarrhea*

FISH

PHOSPHORUS	*Salty fish mainly*

HOT

DRINKS

GRAPHITES	*Disgust*
LACHESIS MUTUS	*Sometimes by paradoxical dysphagia*
PHOSPHORUS	*Tea and hot drinks*
PULSATILLA	*Prefers cold, sweet and refreshing drinks*
SILICEA	

FOODS

BRYONIA	
CHINA (CINCHONA)	*Even though no colic or diarrhea is triggered*
GRAPHITES	*Cooked and hot foods*

PHOSPHORUS	
PULSATILLA	*Likes fresh, spicy, sweet foods*
SILICEA	*Likes fruity and juicy foods*

MILK Pure

CALCAREA CARBONICA	*Badly tolerated, sometimes, but frequent craving in the young adult*
CARBO VEGETABILIS	*As for all fatty foods*
NATRUM CARBONICUM	*Poorly tolerated, diarrhea*
SEPIA	*Same as above*
SILICEA	*Even to breast milk, but this is also an intolerance*

ODOR and SIGHT OF FOOD

ARSENICUM ALBUM	*Cooking odors*
COCCULUS INDICUS	*Fish and grease*
COLCHICUM AUTUMNALE	*Very pronounced hypersensitivity to odors, disgust and nausea mostly for fish and eggs*
IPECA (IPECAC)	*During digestive disorders, disgust for any food leads to nausea and vomiting*
SEPIA	*Cannot stand the sight or smell of food and cooking. Frequent symptom, mostly during pregnancy, sometimes aversion to all foods*

OYSTERS

PHOSPHORUS

SALT

GRAPHITES	*Sometimes*
NATRUM MURIATICUM	*When he is sick of it, sometimes*
PHOSPHORUS	*Craving for salt and salty foods but rejects salty fish and oysters*

STRANGE FOODS

ARSENICUM ALBUM	*Caution and suspicion. Very characteristic*
LYCOPODIUM	*Caution and suspicion. Very characteristic*

SUGAR, sweets

CAUSTICUM	
GRAPHITES	*Frequent, but opposite also exists*

WATER

CAUSTICUM	*Likes all cold drinks except water*

SLEEP

Sleep symptoms are part of the general signs. They are high-value symptoms mainly when spontaneously expressed by patients. Sleep symptoms are valid for sleep and all its epiphenomena but these symptoms are of unequal value. Some are objective, described by patients or family, such as positions, screaming, bruxomania (teeth grinding), sleepwalking; others are subjective, like dreaming.

Readers should be forewarned about the reliability of dreams. A dream is only characteristic if it repeats itself over and over. A medicine is rarely prescribed only on the recurring theme of a dream. In literature, examples of medicines chosen on the sole basis of a dream are purely anecdotal. The most frequent themes, with rare exceptions, do not always have a corresponding medicine. Certain dreams like death, suffocation, and burglary are reliable; others can cautiously be taken into account only as additions to the patients' symptoms and clinical state. Readers should go back to the repertories if they hear an extraordinary dream reported by a patient. The goal of this Memento is to be practical above all, and not to be exhaustive. This explains the brevity of this chapter.

We did not include everything about sleep in this chapter. An important characteristic such as sweating when sleeping is not part of it. The important sign is sweating, and sleep is only a modality, so readers should return to the Chapter "Sweating", under the heading "Going to sleep". This is true for this entire book: readers should return to the appropriate chapter when a specific symptom is not found in one given chapter.

AGGRAVATION (By sleep)

LACHESIS MUTUS	*General aggravation*
NUX VOMICA	*Prolonged sleep*

AGITATED (Sleep)

ACONITUM	
ARGENTUM NITRICUM	*Anxiety due to anticipation*
ARNICA	*Physical overexertion, post-surgery, with sensation of bed too hard*
ARSENICUM ALBUM	*Anxiety, asthma, between 1 and 3 a.m.*
AURUM METALLICUM	*Bone pain*
BELLADONNA	*Congestive headache*
CHINA (CINCHONA)	*Patient weakened by loss of vital fluids, profuse sweating, hyperideation*
CINA	*Infestation with worms (ascarides and oxyurids), bruxomania, frights, coughing, need to snack*
COFFEA TOSTA	*With physical and mental excitation*
HYOSCYAMUS	

KALIUM BROMATUM	*Trembling hands, frights, sleepwalking, coughing*
LACHESIS MUTUS	*Menopause, suffocating sensation*
LYCOPODIUM	*Digestive disorders, chronic nasal obstruction, snoring*
MERCURIUS SOLUBILIS	*Intolerance to the heat of the bed, sweating, salivation*
NUX VOMICA	*With headache and coated tongue when waking up, 3 a.m. awake*
OPIUM	*Due to noise, light sleep never turning into deep sleep*
PHOSPHORUS	*Continuous dreaming, palpitations when lying on the left side*
RHUS TOXICODENDRON	*Sore muscles improved by moving; dreams about daily routine*
SILICEA	*Startled at the slightest noise, awakens at the slightest noise*
STRAMONIUM	*Night frights*
SULFUR (SULPHUR)	*But doesn't complain*
SULFUR IODATUM (SULPHUR IODATUM)	
THUYA (THUJA OCCIDENTALIS)	*At the end of the night, nightmares of falling, death and disease*

BRUXOMANIA

ARSENICUM ALBUM	
BELLADONA	
CHAMOMILLA	
CINA	
COFFEA TOSTA	
HYOSCYAMUS	
IGNATIA	
KALIUM BROMATUM	
PODOPHYLLUM	*Teething*
STRAMONIUM	
SULFUR	
TUBERCULINUM	
ZINCUM METALLICUM	

CHOKING feeling when waking up

GRINDELIA
LACHESIS MUTUS

COMATOSE

ANTIMONIUM TARTARICUM	*Respiratory congestion*
BELLADONNA	*With fever and red face*
GELSEMIUM	*With fever and dark red face*
NUX MOSCHATA	*Falls asleep as soon as activities stop*
OPIUM	*With hot sweating*
STRAMONIUM	

CRIES during sleep

AURUM METALLICUM	*Cries when sleeping, mostly infants*
CHAMOMILLA	*Teething*
CINA	*Worms*
KALIUM BROMATUM	

DEEP

NUX MOSCHATA
NUX VOMICA
OPIUM
PULSATILLA

DREAMS

ACCIDENTS

ARSENICUM ALBUM
GRAPHITES
NUX VOMICA

BURGLARS

ALUMINA	
MAGNESIA CARBONICA	
NATRUM MURIATICUM	*Needs to check*
SILICEA	
ZINCUM METALLICUM	

BURIAL

LACHESIS MUTUS

DEAD bodies

ALUMINA
ANACARDIUM ORIENTALE
ARSENICUM ALBUM
CALCAREA CARBONICA
CROTALUS
GRAPHITES
KALIUM CARBONICUM
LACHESIS MUTUS
MAGNESIA CARBONICA
PHOSPHORUS
SULFUR (SULPHUR)
THUYA (THUJA OCCIDENTALIS)
When patient sleeps on the left side

DEATH (Of)

CALCAREA CARBONICA
LACHESIS MUTUS
SULFUR (SULPHUR)

EFFORTS, Exercise

ARSENICUM ALBUM
RHUS TOXICODENDRON

FALLING from a high place

DIGITALIS
KREOSOTUM
SULFUR (SULPHUR)
THUYA (THUJA OCCIDENTALIS)

NIGHTMARES

ETHYLICUM
KALIUM BROMATUM
LACHESIS MUTUS
STRAMONIUM
SULFUR (SULPHUR)
TARENTULA HISPANICA
THUYA (THUJA OCCIDENTALIS)

SNAKES

ARGENTUM NITRICUM
LAC CANINUM
LACHESIS MUTUS

URINATING

KREOSOTUM
SEPIA
SULFUR (SULPHUR)

ENURESIA

BELLADONA
CAUSTICUM
KALIUM BROMATUM
LYCOPODIUM — *Sometimes over a long period of time*
NATRUM MURIATICUM
PULSATILLA
SEPIA
SILICEA

IMPROVEMENT (By sleep)

NUX VOMICA — *Short nap*
PHOSPHORICUM ACIDUM

PHOSPHORUS
SEPIA

INSOMNIA

ALTITUDE (Due to)

ARSENICUM ALBUM
COCA

ANTICIPATION (Due to)

ARGENTUM NITRICUM	*Physical agitation*
GELSEMIUM	*In spite of feeling sleepy*
IGNATIA	*Sighs*

ANXIETY (Due to)

See **EMOTIONS (Caused by)**

BED (After going to)

AMBRA GRISEA	*Falls asleep in front of the TV and can't sleep when returning to bed*

COLD (Due to a sensation of) feet

CALCAREA CARBONICA
CARBO VEGETABILIS
NITRICUM ACIDUM
PHOSPHORUS
PULSATILLA
SEPIA
SILICEA

DIGESTIVE (Due to digestive disorders)

KALIUM CARBONICUM
LYCOPODIUM
NUX VOMICA

EFFORT Intellectual (After an)

ARSENICUM ALBUM
COFFEA TOSTA
HYOSCYAMUS
LACHESIS MUTUS
NUX VOMICA

EMOTIONS (Caused by)

AMBRA GRISEA	*Broods on problems*
ARGENTUM NITRICUM	*Sense of foreboding*
ARSENICUM ALBUM	*Due to anxiety*

COCCULUS	*Due to anxiety*
COFFEA TOSTA	*Joy, excitation*
HYOSCYAMUS	*Jealousy*
IGNATIA	*Sorrow and upset*
LACHESIS MUTUS	*Jealousy*
NATRUM MURIATICUM	
NUX VOMICA	*Anger*
OPIUM	*After emotion and fear or auditive hypersensitivity*
PULSATILLA	*Affective loss: object or person*
Exciting emotions	
AMBRA GRISEA	*By excitation and being hyper-emotional*
COFFEA TOSTA	*Happy excitation, hyperideation*
HYOSCYAMUS	
NUX VOMICA	*Active and quick-tempered person*

FALLING ASLEEP (While)

AMBRA GRISEA	*Sleep vanishes when subject goes to bed*
ARGENTUM NITRICUM	*Afraid of not sleeping*
CHAMOMILLA	*Pain, teething*
COCCULUS	*After jet lag or perturbation of the sleep cycle*
COFFEA TOSTA	*Hyperideation, happy excitation*
GELSEMIUM	*Apprehension and sleepiness*
GRINDELIA	*Feels suffocated when sleeping*
IGNATIA	*Sorrow*
LACHESIS MUTUS	*Nocturnal hyperactivity, feels suffocated when falling asleep*
LYCOPODIUM	
NATRUM MURIATICUM	*Sorrow, deception*
NUX VOMICA	*With need to sleep in the morning*
OPIUM	*Hypersensitivity to noise*
PULSATILLA	*Thinks about the same idea over and over*
STAPHYSAGRIA	*Ruminates repressed grievances*
SUMBUL	*Brain excitation*
VALERIANA	*Neurotony subject*

FATIGUE (Due to)

ARNICA	*Muscle fatigue*
ARSENICUM ALBUM	*Exhausted patient*
NUX VOMICA	*Nervous fatigue*
RHUS TOXICODENDRON	*Muscle fatigue*

FATIGUE (Due to intellectual)

ALFALFA	*After an infectious disease*
KALIUM PHOSPHORICUM	*Exhausted student*
NUX VOMICA	*Overexertion with irritability*
PHOSPHORICUM ACIDUM	*Exhausted and intellectual indifference*
ZINCUM METALLICUM	*Fidgety legs, restlessness of the lower limbs*

FEAR (Due to)

Of the dark or of being alone

ARSENICUM ALBUM
CAUSTICUM
PHOSPHORUS
STRAMONIUM

Of the night

ARSENICUM ALBUM	*Afraid of death and of the night*
CAUSTICUM	*By anxiety or fear of being alone*
LUESINUM (SYPHILINUM)	*Because of intense bone pains*
PHOSPHORUS	*Fear of being alone*
PULSATILLA	*Needs to be reassured, cuddled*

Of burglars

ARSENICUM ALBUM
NATRUM MURIATICUM

HEAT (Because of a sensation of)

FLUORICUM ACIDUM
PULSATILLA

HEAT of the bed (Because of the)

MERCURIUS SOLUBILIS
SULFUR (SULPHUR)

HEAT of the feet (Because of the)

CALCAREA FLUORICA
CHAMOMILLA
FLUORICUM ACIDUM
MEDORRHINUM
PULSATILLA
SULFUR (SULPHUR)

HOT FLASHES (Due to)

LACHESIS MUTUS
SANGUINARIA
SEPIA

HUMILIATION (After)

AURUM METALLICUM
STAPHYSAGRIA

HUNGER (Due to)

CHINA (CINCHONA)
LYCOPODIUM
PETROLEUM
PHOSPHORUS
PSORINUM
TUBERCULINUM

HYPERSENSITIVITY Auditive (Due to)

ASARUM EUROPAEUM	
CHINA (CINCHONA)	*Asthenic subject*
NUX VOMICA	*Quick-tempered subject*
OPIUM	*With sleepiness*
PHOSPHORUS	*Passionate and empathic subject*

IDEA (The same one) continually returns

CALCAREA CARBONICA
COFFEA TOSTA
GRAPHITES
NATRUM MURIATICUM
PULSATILLA

IDEAS (Due to too many ideas)

AMBRA GRISEA	*Ruminates on problems*
ARGENTUM NITRICUM	*Sense of foreboding*
ARSENICUM ALBUM	*Anxious, afraid of dying*
COFFEA TOSTA	*Lots of ideas, with a happy mood*
LACHESIS MUTUS	*Jealousy*
NUX VOMICA	*Thinks about own multiple projects*
PULSATILLA	*Gentle person who cries easily*

JEALOUSY

HYOSCYAMUS
LACHESIS MUTUS

JOY

COFFEA TOSTA
HYOSCYAMUS

NIGHT (One) out of two

ARSENICUM ALBUM

NOISE (At the slightest)

COFFEA TOSTA
NUX VOMICA
OPIUM

RESTLESSNESS of the lower limbs

CAUSTICUM	*Paretic or rheumatic*
KALIUM CARBONICUM	*Asthenic, dyspeptic and dyspneic*
MEDORRHINUM	*Rheumatic with a burning sensation on the soles of the feet*
ZINCUM METALLICUM	*With intolerance to wine*
ZINCUM VALERIANICUM	*If ZINCUM METALLICUM fails*

SLEEPINESS (With daytime)

BELLADONNA	*Congestive headache*
CALCAREA CARBONICA	
CHAMOMILLA	*Fussy, improved when cradled*
GELSEMIUM	*Afraid of not falling asleep*
LACHESIS MUTUS	*Suffocates as soon as falling asleep*
NUX VOMICA	*Much improved by a short nap*
OPIUM	*Auditive hypersensitivity*
PHOSPHORICUM ACIDUM	*Nervous exhaustion*
PHOSPHORUS	*Anxious, tall and lank, asthenic*
PULSATILLA	*Person who cries easily*
STRAMONIUM	*Afraid of the dark and of being alone*
SULFUR (SULPHUR)	*Cannot stand the heat of the bed*

SORROW, Death (Following)

IGNATIA
NATRUM MURIATICUM
PHOSPHORICUM ACIDUM
SEPIA

STAYING UP Late (After)

COCCULUS

STIMULANTS (Due to)

COFFEA TOSTA
NUX VOMICA

TIMETABLE (According to the)

Before midnight

CHAMOMILLA	*From 9 p.m. to midnight*
CHINA (CINCHONA)	*One day out of two*

See also **FALLING ASLEEP**

After midnight

ACONITUM
ARSENICUM ALBUM
KALIUM BROMATUM
KALIUM CARBONICUM

2 a.m.

SULFUR (SULPHUR)

3 or 4 a.m.

KALIUM BROMATUM
KALIUM CARBONICUM
NUX VOMICA
THUYA (THUJA OCCIDENTALIS)
TUBERCULINUM

5 a.m.

SULFUR (SULPHUR)	*With diarrhea*

At dawn

SEPIA

TOTAL

LUESINUM (SYPHILINUM)

TROUBLES Real or imagined

AMBRA GRISEA	*Broods on bad thoughts*
GELSEMIUM	*Sense of foreboding*
HYOSCYAMUS	*Jealousy*
NATRUM MURIATICUM	*Sorrow*

WAKING UP (After)

AMBRA GRISEA
ARSENICUM ALBUM
BELLADONNA
LACHESIS MUTUS
MERCURIUS SOLUBILIS
NATRUM MURIATICUM
NUX VOMICA
PHOSPHORUS
SEPIA
SILICEA
SULFUR (SULPHUR)

WINE (After drinking)

NUX VOMICA

JOLTS when falling asleep or when sleeping (Woken up by)

ARSENICUM ALBUM
BISMUTHUM
CINA
HYOSCYAMUS
KALIUM CARBONICUM
LACHESIS MUTUS
NATRUM MURIATICUM
PHYSOSTIGMA
PULSATILLA
SILICEA

LACK of sleep, staying up late (After)

COCCULUS	*Dizziness, headaches, nausea*
KALIUM PHOSPHORICUM	*Difficulties in concentrating and memorizing*
PHOSPHORICUM ACIDUM	*Asthenia, indifference, hair loss*
SELENIUM	*Asthenia worse in the summer heat, seborrhea*

LAUGHS in sleep

HYOSCYAMUS
KALIUM BROMATUM
LYCOPODIUM
SILICEA
STRAMONIUM

NAP Long (Aggravation due to)

BRYONIA
LACHESIS MUTUS
LYCOPODIUM
PULSATILLA
STAPHYSAGRIA
SULFUR (SULPHUR)

NEED TO SLEEP FOR A LONG TIME

NATRUM MURIATICUM
PHOSPHORUS

NIGHT FRIGHTS

BORAX	*Jumps at the slightest noise*
CINA	*Worms*
KALIUM BROMATUM	*Aggravation at 3 a.m.*
KALIUM PHOSPHORICUM	
STRAMONIUM	*Aggravation before midnight, needs light*
ZINCUM METALLICUM	*Wakes up screaming; restlessness of the lower limbs*

NOT RESTFUL

AGARICUS MUSCARIUS
ARNICA
ARSENICUM ALBUM
COCCULUS
LACHESIS MUTUS
LUESINUM (SYPHILINUM)
MAGNESIA CARBONICA
MAGNESIA MURIATICUM
NATRUM MURIATICUM
NITRICUM ACIDUM
NUX VOMICA
PHOSPHORUS
PULSATILLA
RHUS TOXICODENDRON
SULFUR (SULPHUR)

POSITION when sleeping or falling asleep

ABDOMEN (Flat on the)

ARSENICUM
BELLADONNA
BRYONIA
CINA
COLOCYNTHIS
LYCOPODIUM
MEDORRHINUM
PODOPHYLLUM
STRAMONIUM

CUDDLED or rocked

CHAMOMILLA *Teething*
KREOSOTUM *Teething*

FETAL position (Genu-pectoral)

ARSENICUM ALBUM
CALCAREA PHOSPHORICA
CINA
LYCOPODIUM
MEDORRHINUM
PHOSPHORUS

HANDS above or below the head

NUX VOMICA
PULSATILLA

HANDS crossed over the abdomen

PULSATILLA

LEGS crossed

RHODODENDRON

LEGS wide open

CHAMOMILLA
PLATINA

LYING on the back

BRYONIA
IGNATIA
LYCOPODIUM
NUX VOMICA
PULSATILLA
RHUS TOXICODENDRON

LYING on the left side

BARYTA CARBONICA
BORAX
LYCOPODIUM
MAGNESIA MURIATICA
SABINA
SANGUINARIA

LYING on the right side

LACHESIS MUTUS
NATRUM SULFURICUM
PHOSPHORUS
SEPIA

SITTING

ARSENICUM ALBUM	*Asthma or cardiac problems*
AURUM METALLICUM	*Cardiac pain*
KALIUM CARBONICUM	*Asthma*

PRURITUS (During sleep)

MERCURIUS SOLUBILIS	*Dermatosis*
MEZEREUM	*Dermatosis*
PSORINUM	*Dermatosis*
PULSATILLA	*Circulatory disorders, venous insufficiency*
SULFUR (SULPHUR)	*Dermatosis*

RHYTHMIC MOVEMENTS (Falling asleep)

CINA
MEDORRHINUM
TUBERCULINUM

SCREAMING during sleep

BORAX
CHAMOMILLA
CINA
LYCOPODIUM
PULSATILLA
STRAMONIUM
ZINCUM METALLICUM

SLEEPINESS Daytime

AMMONIUM CARBONICUM *With daytime obsession*
NUX MOSCHATA
OPIUM

SLEEPING PILLS (Aggravation due to)

BELLADONNA
CHAMOMILLA
COFFEA TOSTA
HYOSCYAMUS
LACHESIS MUTUS
LYCOPODIUM
NUX VOMICA
OPIUM
PULSATILLA
SEPIA
VALERIANA

SLEEPWALKING

KALIUM BROMATUM
KALIUM PHOSPHORICUM
NATRUM MURIATICUM
PHOSPHORUS
SILICEA

TALKS during sleep

BELLADONNA	*Red face*
CINA	*Worms*
HYOSCYAMUS	*Mumbles*
KALIUM BROMATUM	*Often with nightmares and waking up at 3 a.m.*
NATRUM MURIATICUM	*Extremely silent in the daytime*
PULSATILLA	*Frequent*
SEPIA	
SILICEA	
SULFUR (SULPHUR)	
ZINCUM METALLICUM	

WAKING UP LATE

ANACARDIUM ORIENTALE	
CALCAREA CARBONICA	
CALCAREA PHOSPHORICA	
CAUSTICUM	
GRAPHITES	
LACHESIS MUTUS	
LYCOPODIUM	*Irritability and migraine*
MAGNESIA MURIATICA	
NATRUM CARBONICUM	
NUX VOMICA	
PHOSPHORICUM ACIDUM	
PHOSPHORUS	
SEPIA	
SULFUR (SULPHUR)	

WOKEN UP as after a fright

BELLADONNA
BISMUTHUM
BORAX
CHINA (CINCHONA)
KALIUM CARBONICUM
LACHESIS MUTUS
LYCOPODIUM
NATRUM MURIATICUM
NUX VOMICA
PULSATILLA
SEPIA
SPONGIA
SULFUR (SULPHUR)

WOKEN UP because of dreams

ARNICA
BELLADONNA
CHAMOMILLA
HEPAR SULFUR
LACHESIS MUTUS
MERCURIUS SOLUBILIS
NUX VOMICA
PHOSPHORICUM ACIDUM
SULFUR (SULPHUR)

WOKEN UP by hunger

See **INSOMNIA due to HUNGER**

YAWNING

ANTIMONIUM TARTARICUM	*After coughing*
CINA	*Frequent in daytime*
IGNATIA	
IPECA (IPECAC)	*After coughing*
KREOSOTUM	*After coughing*
NUX VOMICA	*During the day*
PULSATILLA	*Before menstruation*

KEYNOTES

A question arose when we wrote this chapter: how can we define the term "keynotes" or key symptoms when, according to the authors, two types of concepts correspond to the same terminology.

For example Adolph von LIPPE, who wrote *Keynotes prescribers*, focused on the most singular symptoms, either by their rarity or their peculiarity, or by their grouping. For him and his followers, these symptoms helped reveal the medicines to prescribe.

The explanation for the term "Keynotes" is completely different for homeopaths in other books where this notion extends to include all the characteristic symptoms of a medicine. This is the case, for example, of *Leaders in the homoeopathic therapeutics* by E.-B. NASH or *Keynotes and characteristics of the materia medica with nosodes* by H.-C. ALLEN.

In recent or contemporary French writings the same duality exists.

The adepts of the first definition - rare and peculiar symptoms - are, for example, D. DEMARQUE, M. CONAN MERIADEC (for whom, furthermore "*A keynote is a characteristic symptom of a medicine because it only exists in the pathogenesis of this medicine*"), J. LAMOTHE ("*A keynote corresponds to a single remedy, or to less than three, or to many remedies but of which only one represents at least 75% of the cases encountered in practice*") or, earlier on, H. DUPRAT.

The adepts of the second proposal - all the characteristic symptoms of a medicine - are represented, for example, by R. SEROR (for whom "*Keynotes are the main symptoms of HERING's high degree, clinically verified*"). This has given rise to a short materia medica where each medicine is presented in six to fifteen lines.

We can then note that: the definition of the term "keynote" differs depending on whether it is used as a singular or plural. This is why "keynotes" of a medicine can constitute a summarized and valorized materia medica. However "the" keynote, being rare, peculiar or important, strongly evokes a particular medicine, and leads physicians to search if a patient exhibits other symptoms of this medicine, before prescribing.

Given these two options, for this chapter we chose to use the "singular", and the definition of D. DEMARQUE: "*Keynotes (meaning symptoms peculiar by nature) are a category of highly characteristic general and local symptoms since they refer to very few medicines, sometimes just one*".

Once his definition was chosen, there were two ways of presenting this chapter:

- either by listing keynote symptoms by categories, with each followed by one or more corresponding medicines. However the choice of the keyword introducing the keynote, and the fact that one keynote could be listed in various categories, proved difficult for reading purposes;
- or by an alphabetical listing of medicines followed by one or more keynotes which are particularly characteristic of that medicine.

We chose the second solution, keeping in mind that this chapter will rarely be used during consultation, but rather will be studied when the reader has time. It is also obvious that not all the medicines from the materia medica are linked to reliable-enough keynotes. This is why the list hereafter is relatively short and certain frequently-used medicines are not part of it.

ABIES NIGRA	*Sensation of hard-boiled egg stuck in the cardia*
ABROTANUM	*Lower body weight loss in spite of good appetite*
ACONITUM NAPELLUS	*Brutal onset of symptoms* *Panic attack* *Aggravation due to or following extreme temperatures (cold or heat)*
ACTAEA RACEMOSA (CIMICIFUGA)	*Pathology proportional to the blood flow during menstruation (dysmenorrhea, headaches, rheumatism)* *Stiffness and sensitivity to pressure, of muscular origin, in an area between the third cervical vertebra to the third dorsal vertebra*
ACTAEA SPICATA	*Painful knuckle deformation*
AESCULUS HIPPOCASTANUM	*Sensation of needles in the rectum (hemorrhoids)*
AETHUSA CYNAPIUM	*For infants, intolerance to milk, vomited immediately after ingestion*
AGARICUS MUSCARIUS	*Sensation of ice needles (facial neuralgia, chilblains)*
AILANTHUS GLANDULOSA	*Sore throat or pharyngitis not reacting to antibiotics*
ALLIUM CEPA	*Corrosive nasal discharge and slight eye-watering*
ALLIUM SATIVUM	*Digestive disorders in big meat eaters*
ALOE SOCOTRINA	*Sphincter insecurity when passing gas or urinating*
ALUMINA	*Dryness of the skin and all mucous membranes* *Soft stool only expelled after prolonged effort*
AMBRA GRISEA	*Insomnia: the urge to sleep disappears when head hits the pillow*
AMMONIUM CARBONICUM	*Dry and plugged-up nose when lying down, at 3 a.m.*
AMMONIUM MURIATICUM	*Sciatic pain aggravated when sitting* *Sensation of tendons being too short*

ANACARDIUM ORIENTALE	*Contradictory impulsions, dual personality: the patient seems to be the victim of a divided will. All symptoms are improved by eating: stomach ache, nausea (mostly pregnancy), headaches, general condition*
ANAGALLIS ARVENSIS	*Aspect of palmar and digital dyshidrosis*
ANGUSTURA VERA	*Stiffness of the lower limbs with need to stretch*
ANTIMONIUM CRUDUM	*Tongue with thick white coating, like milk or chalk (after eating too much)* *Hyperkeratosis* *The child cannot bear to be looked at, touched or carried*
ANTIMONIUM TARTARICUM	*Abundant and viscous pulmonary mucus, very difficult expectoration* *Fluttering of the nostrils (hypoxia)*
APIS MELLIFICA	*Pinkish-red edema, burning and stinging, of the skin, mucous or serous membranes* *Improved by cold wraps*
ARALIA RACEMOSA	*Coughing when lying down*
ARANEA DIADEMA	*Sensation of hand swelling* *Neuralgia with numbness in the cubital area* *Sensitive to humidity*
ARGENTUM METALLICUM	*Sensation of wounded larynx*
ARGENTUM NITRICUM	*Sensation of a splinter stuck in the affected mucous membrane (eyes, larynx, stomach, urethra)* *Noisy and frequent eructation* *Anticipation anxiety, with precipitation*
ARNICA MONTANA	*Sensation of bruising, sore muscles, muscle pains; sensation that the bed is too hard*
ARSENICUM ALBUM	*Sensation of intense burning improved by heat (eye-watering, nasal discharge, earache, pharyngitis, pyrosis and gastralgia, diarrhea, dermatosis and neuralgia)* *Food poisoning* *"Elephant skin"* *Meticulous (telltale sign)*
ARSENICUM IODATUM	*Lichen-like or squamous dermatosis*

ARUM TRIPHYLLUM	*Violent pruritus of the mucous membranes (nose, lips, palate, throat, tongue). Continuously bites lips, and tears off skin until it bleeds, in spite of the pain.* *Voice changes, when speaking louder or singing*
ARUNDO DONAX	*Pruritus of the ear canal if allergic coryza*
ASA FOETIDA	*Esophageal anti-peristalsis and sensation of a pharyngeal lump* *Difficult and noisy eructation*
ASARUM EUROPAEUM	*Intolerance to the slightest noise due to nervous hypersensitivity*
ASCLEPIAS TUBEROSA	*Pains around lowest intercostal spaces on left, pleurisy or neuralgia*
AURUM METALLICUM	*Sensation of heart stopping, following a violent shock*
BARYTA CARBONICA	*At the doctor's, the child hides, or hides behind hands, looks through fingers, in a context of mental or affective retardation, or excessive shyness*
BELLADONNA	*Inflammatory and congestive phenomena with sensorial hypersensitivity*
BELLIS PERENNIS	*Breast and pelvic trauma*
BENZOÏCUM ACIDUM	*Dark brown ammonia-smelling urine, "like horse urine"*
BERBERIS VULGARIS	*Centrifugal radiating pain (kidney, bladder or other areas)*
BORAX	*Fear of bending over, or downward movement (stairs, elevators, planes, swings, boats, etc.)*
BOTHROPS LANCEOLATUS	*Black-blood flow due to disseminated intra-vascular coagulation. Clinical context more intense than CROTALUS*
BOVISTA GIGANTEA	*Headaches with sensation of swelling of the head and hands*
BROMUM	*Respiratory disorders improved at sea or at the seaside*
BRYONIA ALBA	*Improvement by total immobility and strong pressure on the problem area (headaches, cough, mastitis, joint pains), aggravation at the slightest movement* *Dryness of the mouth with a bitter taste*

CACTUS GRANDIFLORUS	*Constricted sensation, like in a vice*
CALCAREA CARBONICA	*Cold damp feet as if wearing wet stockings (or sensation)* *Cravings for eggs and indigestible foods (chalk, paper, wood, dirt, etc.) in children*
CACAREA FLUORICA	*Chronic lumbar pain after failure of RHUS TOXICODENDRON*
CALCAREA PHOSPHORICA	*Pain in the epiphysis and symphysis*
CANTHARIS VESICATORIA	*Very violent vesical burning, before, during and after urinating; infrequent, scanty urination* *Phlyctena*
CAPSICUM ANNUUM	*Sensation of intense burning of the mucous membranes, "as if pepper was poured on", not improved by heat. Mastoiditis painful when touched*
CARBO ANIMALIS	*Cyanotic rosacea with varicose veins*
CARBO VEGETABILIS	*Need to be fanned (hypoxemia, hypercapnia)*
CARBONEUM SULFURATUM	*Neuralgia with numbness*
CAULOPHYLLUM	*Cervix dystocia with uterine rigidity and inertia*
CAUSTICUM	*Stiffness aggravated by dry cold* *Paresis or paralysis* *Hypersensitive to others' sorrows*
CHAMOMILLA	*Hyperesthesia to pain with irritability, tantrums, violence or rudeness* *Improved by passive movement (rocking movement)*
CHEIRANTHUS	*Pathology or extraction of wisdom teeth*
CHELIDONIUM MAJUS	*Pain at the lower angle of the right scapula (hepatic or pulmonary affection)*
CHIMAPHILA UMBELLATA	*Prostatism (sensation of sitting on a ball) with mucus-containing urine*
CHINA (CINCHONA)	*Exhaustion with loss of fluids (blood, sweat, diarrhea)*
CINA	*Nasal and anal pruritus (helminthiasis)* *Angry when touched or spoken to*

CINNABARIS (MERCURIUS SULPHURATUS RUBER)	*Sensation of painful pressure at the base of the nose, as if wearing heavy glasses*
CLEMATIS ERECTA	*Intermittent urinating, and urine leakage after micturition*
COCA	*High altitude disorders (mountains, hot air balloon)*
COCCULUS INDICUS	*Perturbation of the sleep cycle* *Disorders related to lack of sleep*
COCCUS CACTI	*Cough with expectoration of clear abundant mucus, long and stringy*
COFFEA TOSTA	*Affluence of ideas, day or night*
COLCHICUM	*Hypersensitivity to odors*
COLLINSONIA CANADENSIS	*Constipation and/or hemorrhoids during pregnancy*
COLOCYNTHIS	*Various cramping pains, improved by pressure, heat or bending over*
CONDURANGO	*Fissures on corners of the lips*
CONIUM MACULATUM	*Dizziness worsened when lying down and when turning the head*
CORALLIUM RUBRUM	*Spasmodic cough with red face*
CROTALUS HORRIDUS	*Black blood flowing out of all body orifices; does not coagulate*
CROTON TIGLIUM	*Very intense pruritus improved by soft rubbing*
CUPRUM METALLICUM	*Voluntary or involuntary muscle spasms or cramping*
CYCLAMEN EUROPAEUM	*Ophthalmic migraine with dizziness before or during menstruation periods*
DIOSCOREA VILLOSA	*Paroxysmal visceralgia or neuralgia improved when bending backwards*
DOLICHOS PRURIENS	*Skin pruritus with no lesions*
DROSERA ROTUNDIFOLIA	*Spasmodic dry cough with laryngeal tickling*
DULCAMARA	*Following exposure to damp cold (rain, fog, bath) or catching a cold after sweating or getting wet*

EQUISETUM HIEMALE	*Bladder heaviness not improved by urinating during acute or chronic urinary infections*
EUGENIA JAMBOSA	*Painful acne papules*
EUPATORIUM PERFOLIATUM	*Pain when applying pressure on the eyeballs, in feverish conditions*
EUPHRASIA OFFICINALIS	*Corrosive eye-watering with non-irritant nasal discharge*
FERRUM PHOSPHORICUM	*Low fever with progressive onset, with alternation of paleness and redness of the face* *Painful cough due to tracheitis*
FLUORICUM ACIDUM	*Pruritus on scars*
FRAXINUS AMERICANA	*Menorrhagia on fibroid uterus*
GELSEMIUM SEMPERVIRENS	*Paresis with obsession, shaking and weakness*
GLONOÏNUM	*Throbbing congestion of the head and neck*
GNAPHALIUM POLYCEPHALUM	*Neuralgia with alternation of pain and paresthesia on outside of the thigh*
GRAPHITES	*Honey-like discharges*
GRINDELIA ROBUSTA	*Lying down leads to suffocating dyspnea*
HAMAMELIS VIRGINIANA	*Sensation that veins are bursting*
HEKLA LAVA	*Exostosis*
HELLEBORUS NIGER	*In a state of stupor with oliguria*
HELONIAS DIOÏCA	*Profuse and pruriginous leukorrhea that looks like curdled milk*
HEPAR SULFUR	*Suppuration of the skin and mucous membranes with hypersensitivity to cold, to the touch and to pain*
HYDRASTIS CANADENSIS	*Sticky, thick, yellow discharges of the mucous membranes*
HYOSCYAMUS NIGER	*Obscene or violent delirium*
HYPERICUM PERFORATUM	*Pain following a nerve trajectory*

IGNATIA AMARA	*Mental hypersensitivity with spasms*
IPECA (IPECAC)	*Nausea with clean tongue*
IRIS VERSICOLOR	*Hyperacidity along the digestive tube*
KALIUM ARSENICOSUM	*Cutaneous ARSENICUM ALBUM aggravated by heat*
KALIUM BICHROMICUM	*Greenish-yellow discharges of the mucous membranes* *Skin or mucous membranes ulcerations with clean-cut edges*
KALIUM BROMATUM	*Constant agitation of the hands or fingers*
KALIUM CARBONICUM	*Anxiety like a blow in the pit of the stomach* *Transfixing and erratic pains*
KALIUM IODATUM	*Pains in the facial bones with sensation of "fullness" of the head*
KALIUM MURIATICUM	*Thick white discharges*
KALIUM PHOSPHORICUM	*Alternation of mental exhaustion and hyperactivity with irritability*
KALMIA LATIFOLIA	*Lightening-like neuralgia*
KREOSOTUM	*Foul-smelling and corrosive discharges of the mucous membranes; bleeding at the slightest contact*
LACHESIS MUTUS	*Sensation of constriction with intolerance to any tightness* *Improved by physiological or pathological discharge*
LACHNANTES TINCTORIA	*Cervical pain*
LATRODECTUS MACTANS	*Coronary insufficiency (in addition to the patient being hospitalized and receiving classical treatment)*
LAUROCERASUS	*Choking improved by lying down*
LEDUM PALUSTRE	*Swelling of the joints, pale and cold to the touch, improved by a cold bath*
LILIUM TIGRINUM	*Pelvic heaviness: neurotic "terrain"*
LUESINUM (SYPHILINUM)	*Total insomnia and bone pains aggravated at night*

LYCOPODIUM	*Bad mood when waking up and intolerance to contradiction* *Migraine if meals are eaten late* *Quickly satiated* *Pruritus scratched until it bleeds*
MAGNESIA CARBONICA	*Acrid odor of the body and stools* *Premenstrual rhinopharyngitis*
MAGNESIA MURIATICA	*Hard little stools, like sheep droppings*
MAGNESIA PHOSPHORICA	*Cramping and spasms improved when bent over, or by strong local pressure, or by heat*
MEDORRHINUM	*Diaper rash. Fetal position in children*
MELILOTUS OFFICINALIS	*Pounding headache improved by epistaxis*
MEPHITIS PUTORIUS	*Spasmodic cough with choking*
MERCURIUS CORROSIVUS	*Intense and burning tenesmus (throat, bladder, rectum)*
MERCURIUS CYANATUS	*False membranes*
MERCURIUS SOLUBILIS	*"Goose bumps" on skin surface with suppuration* *Mercurial mouth (tonsils)*
MEZEREUM	*Pain in the upper maxillaries*
MOSCHUS	*Fainting and hysteria-like spasms*
MUREX PURPUREA	*Sensation of the pubic symphysis widening during pregnancy*
MURIATICUM ACIDUM	*Hemorrhoid thrombosis*
MYRISTICA SEBIFERA	*Whitlow*
NAJA NAJA (NAJA TRIPUDIANS)	*Functional or organic precordialgia (mitral valve prolapse (MVP), following a heart attack)*
NATRUM MURIATICUM	*Craving for salt* *Extremely thin upper body* *Introversion*
NATRUM SULFURICUM	*Sensitivity to humidity for all symptoms* *Asthma aggravated by fog*

NITRICUM ACIDUM	*Fissures of the skin and the mucous membranes with clear-cut edges, and a sanious center* *Splinter-like pain* *Golden-yellow aspect of the warts*
NUX MOSCHATA	*Irrepressible sleepiness* *Dryness of the skin and the mucous membranes*
NUX VOMICA	*Spasmodic manifestations* *Hyper-reactivity* *Post-prandial drowsiness improved by a short nap* *Dyspepsia improved by vomiting*
ONOSMODIUM	*Libido drop*
OPIUM	*Severe pathological phenomena with absence of pain*
OXALICUM ACIDUM	*Linear neuralgia with numbness of the extremities*
PAEONIA	*Painful oozing anal fissures*
PALLADIUM	*Right ovary pain*
PAREIRA BRAVA	*Dysuria with spasmodic pain* *Needs to squat to urinate*
PARIS QUADRIFOLIA	*Left facial neuralgia with sensation that the eye is being pulled inwards*
PETROLEUM	*Winter, dirty-looking crevasses and cracking*
PETROSELINUM SATIVUM	*Pain and pruritus in the navicular fossa* *Imperious urge to urinate* *Aggravated by urethral catheterization*
PHELLANDRIUM	*Fetid, abundant expectoration in chronic bronchitis*
PHOSPHORICUM ACIDUM	*Deep asthenia with indifference to everything due to mental overexertion*
PHOSPHORUS	*Hungry when feverish* *Hands are burning hot*
PHYTOLACCA	*Dark redness of the tonsils' anterior pillars* *Dysphagia irradiating up to the ears, with aching muscles*
PLANTAGO MAJOR	*Dental neuralgia*

PLATINA	*Spasmodic manifestations and painful genital hyperesthesia*
PLUMBUM METALLICUM	*Violent cramping neuralgia*
PODOPHYLLUM PELTATUM	*Watery, tiring, explosive diarrhea*
POLYGONUM AVICULARE	*Pain and deformation in the knuckles*
PRUNUS SPINOSA	*Bursting pain in the eyeballs*
PSORINUM	*Sensation of well-being the day before a migraine*
PULSATILLA	*Variable (mood, cough, digestion, transit, discharges, pain, etc.)*
RADIUM BROMATUM	*Pain in the lumbar joints aggravated at the beginning of movement by hypersensitivity to humidity*
RANA BUFO (BUFO RANA)	*Lymphangitis*
RANUNCULUS BULBOSUS	*Intercostal neuralgia improved by slight touch and humidity*
RAPHANUS SATIVUS NIGER	*Confined painful intestinal gas*
RATANHIA	*Anal-rectal pains prolonged a long time after bowel movement*
RHEUM OFFICINALE	*Diarrhea with an acrid odor, after eating green fruit*
RHODODENDRON	*Rheumatoid or neuralgic pain sensitive to stormy weather*
RHUS TOXICODENDRON	*Painful stiffness after resting for a long time, the pain is strong at the beginning of movement and fades as the joints "loosen up"*
ROBINIA	*Intense pyrosis rising into the mouth*
RUMEX CRISPUS	*Coughing when inhaling fresh air*
RUTA GRAVEOLENS	*Tendinous and periosteal trauma*
SABADILLA	*Pruritus of the nasal mucous membranes and soft palate, and compulsive sneezing*
SABINA	*Bright red blood menorrhagia with clotting and pain from the sacrum to the pubis*

SAMBUCUS	*Dyspnea and nasal obstruction with profuse sweating*
SANGUINARIA CANADENSIS	*Weekly migraine on the right side or pounding headache* *Localized redness of the cheeks*
SECALE CORNUTUM	*Intense burning like hot coals improved by cold, with objective coldness of the body* *"ARSENICUM ALBUM seeking cold"*
SENECIO AUREUS	*Amenorrhea with sensation of impending menstrual periods and vicariate phenomena*
SENNA	*Acetone odor to breath*
SEPIA	*Heaviness (cephalic, occipital, gastric, pelvic, genital, lumbar, renal, and "mood")* *General improvement with exertion*
SILICEA	*Chronic suppuration*
SPIGELIA ANTHELMIA	*Violent cephalic neuralgia and headache migrating to the left*
SPONGIA TOSTA	*Croup-like, dry cough*
STANNUM METALLICUM	*Pulmonary congestion with extreme weakness* *Neuralgia beginning and ending progressively*
STAPHYSAGRIA	*Cystalgia with burning between urinations* *Following urogenital traumas*
STICTA PULMONARIA	*Sensation of constriction at the base of the nose*
STRAMONIUM	*High continuous fever with agitation and little pain*
SULFUR (SULPHUR)	*Congestion, redness mostly of the orifices, burns*
SYMPHYTUM	*Following bone and periosteal trauma*
TABACUM	*Nausea with hypersalivation improved by fresh air*
TARENTULA CUBENSIS	*Tendency to phlegmon with infiltration, purple indurations*
TEREBINTHINA	*Dark blood hematuria with oliguria*
THALLIUM METALLICUM	*Iatrogenic alopecia*

THERIDION CURRASSAVICUM	*Dizziness with auditive hypersensitivity (not very reliable)*
THUYA (THUJA OCCIDENTALIS)	*Garlic-smelling sweat* *Sensation as if bones were made of glass* *Soft and breakable nails, with stratification or undulations*
TRILLIUM PENDULUM	*Painful sensation as if the sacroiliac joints and the hips were coming apart, improved by a tight bandage*
TUBERCULINUM	*Agitation and asthenia* *Progressive weight loss in spite of a good and constant appetite*
TUBERCULINUM AVIAIRE	*Fragility of the ENT area, mostly the ear*
TUBERCULINUM RESIDUUM	*Sclerosis and fibrosis of the joints, aponeurotic tissues and the skin* *Stiffness improved by movement, not influenced by hygrometric variations*
URTICA URENS	*Pruritus aggravated when in contact with water and cold wraps*
USTILAGO	*Blackish-blood uterine flow with small clots*
VERATRUM ALBUM	*Cold, profuse sweating*
VERATRUM VIRIDE	*Intense cephalic congestion and red face with slow soft pulse*
VERBASCUM THAPSUS	*Facial neuralgia with sudden crushing pain, aggravated when chewing*
VIPERA REDI	*Inflammatory edema with pain along the vein trajectories, aggravated when dangling legs*
ZINCUM METALLICUM	*Headaches and dizziness aggravated by drinking wine* *Restlessness of the lower limbs with continuous shaking of the legs and feet*

Printed by IMP Alpes
La Roche sur Foron 74800, France
February 2006

Legal deposit : February 2006
Printing N° : 509017

Printed in France